A Text Book Of

COMMUNICATION SKILLS

As Per PCI Regulations

FIRST YEAR B. PHARM.
Semester I

Dr. Meenu Pandey

M.Phil (Eng Lit), M.Ed., M.Lib, PGDTE, PG Dip in Yoga, PGDCA, Ph.D.
Professor,
HOD of Humanities, of LNCT, Bhopal, M.P.

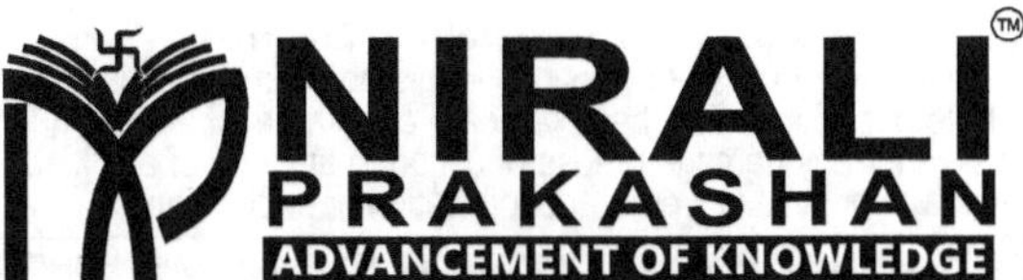

N4010

Fifth Edition : **February 2020**
© : **Author**

Published By :
NIRALI PRAKASHAN
Abhyudaya Pragati, 1312, Shivaji Nagar,
Off J.M. Road, PUNE – 411005
Tel - (020) 25512336/37/39, Fax - (020) 25511379
Email : niralipune@pragationline.com

> ## DISTRIBUTION CENTRES

PUNE

Nirali Prakashan : 119, Budhwar Peth, Jogeshwari Mandir Lane, Pune 411002, Maharashtra
(For orders within Pune)   Tel : (020) 2445 2044, Mobile : 9657703145
Email : niralilocal@pragationline.com

Nirali Prakashan : S. No. 28/27, Dhayari, Near Asian College Pune 411041
(For orders outside Pune)   Tel : (020) 24690204 Fax : (020) 24690316; Mobile : 9657703143
Email : bookorder@pragationline.com

MUMBAI

Nirali Prakashan : 385, S.V.P. Road, Rasdhara Co-op. Hsg. Society Ltd.,
Girgaum, Mumbai 400004, Maharashtra; Mobile : 9320129587
Tel : (022) 2385 6339 / 2386 9976, Fax : (022) 2386 9976
Email : niralimumbai@pragationline.com

> ## DISTRIBUTION BRANCHES

JALGAON

Nirali Prakashan : 34, V. V. Golani Market, Navi Peth, Jalgaon 425001, Maharashtra,
Tel : (0257) 222 0395, Mob : 94234 91860; Email : niralijalgaon@pragationline.com

KOLHAPUR

Nirali Prakashan : New Mahadvar Road, Kedar Plaza, 1st Floor Opp. IDBI Bank, Kolhapur 416 012
Maharashtra. Mob : 9850046155; Email : niralikolhapur@pragationline.com

NAGPUR

Nirali Prakashan : Above Maratha Mandir, Shop No. 3, First Floor,
Rani Jhanshi Square, Sitabuldi, Nagpur 440012, Maharashtra
Tel : (0712) 254 7129; Email : niralinagpur@pragationline.com

DELHI

Nirali Prakashan : 4593/15, Basement, Agarwal Lane, Ansari Road, Daryaganj
Near Times of India Building, New Delhi 110002 Mob : 08505972553
Email : niralidelhi@pragationline.com

BENGALURU

Nirali Prakashan : Maitri Ground Floor, Jaya Apartments, No. 99, 6th Cross, 6th Main,
Malleswaram, Bengaluru 560003, Karnataka; Mob : 9449043034
Email: niralibangalore@pragationline.com

Other Branches : Hyderabad, Chennai

niralipune@pragationline.com | www.pragationline.com
Also find us on f   www.facebook.com/niralibooks

Preface

The objective of this book is to introduce students to the world of communications in a global context and equip them with the communication skills necessary to operate effectively within the corporate world in order to highlight their strengths and promote their potential in an increasingly competitive market. The book provides a strong theoretical foundation of organizational communication for the business and professional communication. Featuring coverage of the most up-to-date skill set available, the book considers the rapid changes in professional communication due to the global economy, advances in information technology, and an increasingly diverse workforce. The authors' engaging narrative style, the unique CCCD model (Choosing, Creating, Coordinating, and Delivering) for building presentation competencies.

The study material in the 'Communication Skills' helps the students to refine their written and verbal communication skills so that they can effectively inform and persuade different readers in different contexts.

Dr. Meenu Pandey

Syllabus

UNIT 1

Communication Skills: Introduction, Definition, The Importance of Communication, The Communication Process-Source, Message, Encoding, Channel, Decoding, Receiver, Feedback, Context

Barriers to Communication: Physiological Barriers, Physical Barriers, Cultural Barriers, Language Barriers, Gender Barriers, Interpersonal Barriers, Psychological Barriers, Emotional Barriers

Perspectives in Communication: Introduction, Visual Perception, Language, Other Factors affecting our perspectives-Past Experiences, Prejudices, Feelings, Environment

UNIT II

Elements of Communication: Introduction, Face to Face Communication, Tone of Voice, Body Language (Non-Verbal Communication), Verbal Communication, Physical Communication

Communication Style: Introduction, The Communication Styles Matrix with example for each – Direct Communication Style, Spirited Communication Style, Systematic Communication Style, Considerate Communication Style

UNIT III

Basic Listening Skills: Introduction, Self-Awareness, Active Listening, Becoming an Active Listener, Listening in Difficult Situations

Effective Written Communication: Introduction, When and When Not to Use Written Communication-Complexity of the Topic, Amount of Discussion Required, Shades of Meaning, Formal Communication

Writing Effectively: Subject Lines, Put the Main Points First, Know Your Audience, Organization of the Message

UNIT IV

Interview Skills: Purpose of an Interview, Do's and Don'ts of an Interview.

Giving Presentations: Dealing with Fears, Planning Your Presentation, Structuring Your Presentation, Delivering Your Presentation, Techniques of Delivery

UNIT V

Group Discussion: Introduction, Communication Skills in Group Discussion, Do's and Don'ts of Group Discussions.

***

CONTENTS

***

Unit I

Chapter ... 1

COMMUNICATION SKILLS

♦ LEARNING OBJECTIVES ♦

Objectives of this chapter are:

- *To make the students aware of basic terms used in communication process*
- *Different elements or components of communication*
- *Different steps of communication process and importance of effective communication.*

1.1 COMMUNICATION

The word communication has been derived from the Latin word 'communicare', which literally means to share, to give and to impart; it means communication is the process of transferring or exchange of information from one source/person to another. It includes facts, emotions, values and feelings. Communication is a continuous process; there may be a time gap but it never stops. Communication is a process of exchanging verbal and non-verbal messages. It is a continuous process. Pre-requisite of communication is a message. This message must be conveyed through some medium to the recipient. It is essential that this message must be understood by the recipient in the same terms as intended by the sender. He must respond within a time frame. Thus, communication is a two-way process and is incomplete without a feedback from the recipient to the sender on how well the message is understood by him.

1.2 DEFINITIONS OF COMMUNICATION

- *"Communication is exchange of facts, ideas, opinion or emotions by two or more persons".*

  – William Newman

- *"Communication is a continuing and thinking process dealing with the transmission and understanding of ideas, facts and courses of action".* **– George and Terry**

> • *"Communication is the process of passing information and understanding from one person to another".*   **– Keith and Davis**
> • *"Communication is the sum of all the things one person does when he wants to create understanding in the mind of another. It is a bridge of meaning. It involves a systematic and continuous process of telling, listening and understanding".*   **– Louis A. Allen**

1.3 CHARACTERISTICS OF COMMUNICATION

Different characteristics of communication are given below:

- Communication is an ongoing process; when communication is absent human activity seizes to exist.
- Communication is essentially a two-way process. Information has not only to be sent but also to be received and understood.
- Communication is essential in all types of organizations and at all levels of management. It pervades all human relationship.
- It consists not only of facts but ideas and emotions too; it can be verbal or nonverbal.
- It is result-oriented; it can be effective if the sender and receiver both are aware of the goal of communication.
- It is a dynamic process.
- It is an interdisciplinary science. Knowledge derived from several sciences is used in communication.

1.4 IMPORTANCE OF EFFECTIVE COMMUNICATION

Communication is important for the following purposes:

- To present yourselves in a better way.
- To develop good interpersonal relation.
- To prove yourself the best amongst all in a highly competitive environment.
- To transfer the information.
- To deal with growing diversity of the business world.
- To deal with complexity of technical information.
- A tool to get a job.
- Essential to job success.
- For motivational counselling and perseverance.
- To impart education.
- To improve discipline.
- To adjust to environment and surroundings.
- To receive messages.
- To provide advice.
- To issue order and instruction.
- To facilitate coordination.
- To establish effective leadership.
- For job satisfaction.
- To develop democratic environment in any organization.

1.5 COMPONENTS OF COMMUNICATION

The main components of the communication process are as follows:

Sender/Encoder: The sender/encoder is a person who sends the message. A sender makes use of symbols (words or graphic or visual aids) to convey the message and produce the required response, for instance, a training manager conducting training for a new batch of employees. Sender may be an individual or a group or an organization. The views, background, approach, skills, competencies, and knowledge of the sender have a great impact on the message. The verbal and non-verbal symbols chosen are essential in ascertaining interpretation of the message by the recipient in the same terms as intended by the sender.

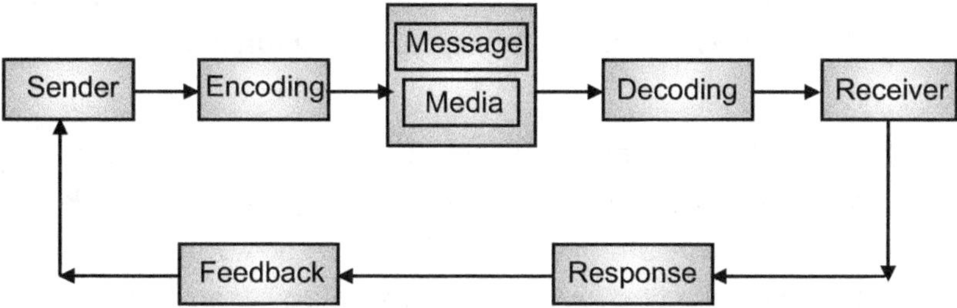

Fig. 1.1: Components of Communication Process

- **Message:** Message is a key idea that the sender wants to communicate. It is a sign that elicits the response of recipient. Communication process begins with deciding about the message to be conveyed. It must be ensured that the main objective of the message is clear.

- **Medium:** Medium is a means used to exchange/transmit the message. The sender must choose an appropriate medium for transmitting the message else the message might not be conveyed to the desired recipients. The choice of appropriate medium of communication is essential for making the message effective and correctly interpreted by the recipient. This choice of communication medium varies depending upon the features of communication. For instance, written medium is chosen when a message has to be conveyed to a small group of people, while an oral medium is chosen when spontaneous feedback is required from the recipient as misunderstandings are cleared then and there.

- **Recipient/Decoder:** The recipient/decoder is a person for whom the message is intended/aimed/targeted. The degree to which the decoder understands the message is dependent upon various factors such as knowledge of recipient, their responsiveness to the message, and the reliance of encoder on decoder.

- **Feedback:** Feedback is the main component of communication process as it permits the sender to analyze the efficacy of the message. It helps the sender in confirming the correct interpretation of message by the decoder. Feedback may be verbal (through words) or non-verbal (in the form of smiles, sighs, etc.). It may take a written form also in the form of memos, reports, etc.

1.6 PROCESS OF COMMUNICATION

The word process suggests that communication exists as a flow through a sequence or series of steps. Communication is an exchange of meaning and understanding. Meaning is central to communication and transfer of meaning is the central objective of communication process. Communication is an interactive process. The communication agents involved in the process of communication are the sender and receiver. Thus we can say communication is a dynamic and interactive process.

There are five steps in the process of communication: **Ideation, Encoding, Transmission, Decoding, and Feedback/Response**

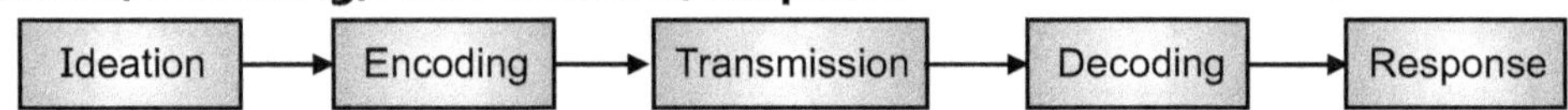

Fig. 1.2: Five Steps of Process of Communication

Ideation: It refers to the formation of an idea or selection of a message to be communicated. The scope of ideation is determined by the sender's knowledge, experiences and abilities as well as the purpose of communication and the context of the communicative situation. Messages generally have two kinds of context – logical and emotional.

Encoding: It is the process of changing information into some form of logical coded message in formal situations. Encoding involves –

- Selecting a language.
- Selecting a medium of communication.
- Selecting an appropriate communicative form.

Selecting a communicative form largely depends upon the sender, receiver relationship and the overall goal of communicative situation. Oral communication may be in the form of face to face communication or face off communication. Written communication may be in the form of reports, letters, e-mails, memorandum, proposals etc.

Transmission: Transmission refers to the flow of message over the chosen channel. Transmission confirms the medium selected during the process of encoding and keeps the communication channel free from interference or noise so that message has reached the receiver without any disturbance. It is also one of the most basic aspects of communications. It also involves choosing the proper place (where to communicate), a proper way (how to communicate) and the time (when to communicate). For communication to be effective it is essential that the right time, the right place and the right method is chosen.

Decoding: It is the process of converting a message into thoughts by translating the received stimuli into interpreted meaning in order to understand the message communicated. It is important to note that it is the message that is transferred from one person to another. The receiver has to assign the message in order to understand it. The process of decoding involves interpretation and analysis of a message. Decoding in oral communication includes listening and understanding and in written communication it refers to reading and understanding a written message. Effective decoding is very important for a successful communication as any misinterpretation of a message may lead to confusion and misunderstanding.

Response/Feedback: It is the action and reaction of receiver to the message. It has the sender to know that the message was received and understood. It is the key to communication as the effectiveness of communication depends on how congruent a receiver's response is with the meaning intended by the sender. Immediate answer of any question is known as response while answer given after a time lag is known as feedback.

Importance of Feedback in Communication

Feedback is very important part of a communication. In any organization feedback can play a very positive role in the development of the organization. The success and failure of the message depends upon the feedback only. Feedback is the reaction of the attempts or the efforts being taken by the organizations or any individual.

The response of the receiver that is sent back to the source forms a feedback. It helps the source/sender to know that the message was received correctly. A good strategy of giving feedback is to follow a three-tier process –

* Listen to what the sender is trying to communicate
* Repeat the central idea of message to ensure that your intention has brightly been understood
* Finally, give a response
* Feedback should not be repeated

Communication Situation

The communication situation is said to exist when –

* There is a person (sender or transmitter) desirous of passing on some information
* There is another person (receiver) to whom the information is to be passed on
* The receiver partly or wholly understands the message passed on to him
* The receiver responds to the message, that is, there is some kind of feedback.

The communication situation cannot exist in the absence of any of these four components. Two gentlemen greeting each other with folded hands constitute a communication situation, for

(a) There is a person desirous of sending a message (greeting).
(b) There is another person to receive this message.
(c) When the first person folds his hands, the second one understands that he is being greeted and
(d) The second person immediately responds back by folding his own hands.

But if a Hindi speaking person addresses a French speaking person in Hindi, the communication situation does not exist, for though there is a person desirous of sending a message, the message is not understood and consequently there is no feedback.

EXERCISE

Answer the following questions:

1. What do you understand by communication?
2. What do you understand by sender?
3. What do you understand by encoding?
4. What do you understand by feedback?
5. Discuss the characteristics of communication.
6. Discuss the essentials of communication.
7. Discuss the limitations of communication.
8. Discuss the importance of communication.
9. How can communication skills help in the growth of an organization?
10. What do you understand by the process of communication?
11. Define cycle of communication. Discuss role of feedback in the cycle of communication.
12. Discuss the role of a sender in the process of communication. What can a sender do to the right message?
13. How can you minimize the communication gap between the sender and the receiver?
14. Draw and explain the process of communication.
15. What are the steps of communication process? Describe in detail.
16. How is feedback important in communication? Give two examples of delayed feedback.

Chapter ... 2

BARRIERS TO COMMUNICATION

◆ LEARNING OBJECTIVES ◆

Objectives of this chapter are:

- *to make the students learn about different types of hindrances caused in free flow of message from sender to receiver.*
- *to make them understand about different interpersonal and intrapersonal barriers, physical and biological barriers, physical and psychological barriers and different linguistic barriers.*
- *to provide different ways to overcome these barriers.*

2.1 INTRODUCTION

Communication is a complex communicative process, involving shared assumptions and unspoken agreement between individuals. It is just like a nervous system of an enterprise. It serves as the lubricant, fostering the smooth operation of management process. Thus, it is very essential to maintain an effective and efficient flow of communication in all directions. There may occur frequent errors and misunderstanding in communication; due to them the message received is not complete or we can say it becomes distorted or truncated. Barriers are the obstacles which prevent us from transmitting our ideas meaningfully. Barriers or obstacles or hurdles distort the message and make communication ineffective. The barriers to communication are obstacles in the process of communication. In fact we cannot remove them from communication, but try to minimize them. Some of the important barriers to communication are – physical, personal, psychological, emotional, status, linguistic, semantic, pre-mature evaluation, inattentive listening, conflicting information, loss in transmission, poor retention, disinterest, previous experiences, physical discomfort, referent confusion etc.

(A) Physiological Barriers:

Physiology is the state of the human body and mind. Physiological barriers of communication occur due to the physical condition of sender or receiver which might even be physical disabilities. It includes sensory dysfunction and other physical dysfunctions. Effective communication requires proper functioning of the senses in both the sender and the receiver. Limitation of human body and mind adds up to the physiological barrier causing interruption in message from reaching its destination or having meaning. For example, a person with short-term memory loss is unable to convey the message after a while as he/she forgets the message and hence the communication fails.

2.2 CAUSES OF PHYSIOLOGICAL BARRIERS

1.　**Deafness and Hearing Impairment:** A receiver with hearing impairment or hearing loss cannot receive an audio message. The person also cannot talk with people face to face easily. If the hearing problem is not very severe, he/she might only hear some words and is unable to get the intended meaning out of the message. Similarly, if a sender who is hearing impaired sends a message, the sender won't be able to get feedback. The communication is limited and thus, not effective as with people without hearing difficulties. Hearing problems can be hereditary, developmental or from other conditions. The person might have speech problems incase he/she had hearing problem since birth or small age.

2.　**Blindness and Vision Impairment:** Use of eyes in communication is as important as other parts of body, as formation of message mostly happens by seeing. Loss of vision, vision impediment, myopia (short sightedness), hypermetropia (long sightedness), blurred vision, tunnel vision, etc. are some types of vision impairment. When people cannot see properly, their message is unclear and misses many descriptions. Also the sender cannot predict the mood of the receiver or the body language so the communication is totally ineffective.

3.　**Speech Disorders:** Speech problems are barriers to communication as speech is a tool for communication. There are many kinds of speech disorders like apraxia, cluttering, stuttering, dysarthria, muteness, etc. Some disorders affect fluency of communication whereas some disorders prevent communication altogether. Speech impediments like stuttering and stammering only affect clarity of the message. Whereas apraxia is a speech disorder in which the parts of brain, which control speech, do not work due to damage, many other speech disorders similar to the ones mentioned above disrupt the communication process as they are not able to use proper speech to communicate.

4.　**Memory:** Poor retention is a cause for physiological communication barrier as human memory is limited. The function of the brain is not to remember each and every bit of information but only the ones that the brain thinks will be needed in future. And information in the memory is also not permanent. So it is lost with time. Retention is needed to store information and send true information across to receiver. Poor retention and forgetting information lead to breakdown of communication.

5.　Selective Perception, Filtering and Alertness (Attention): The physiological conditions dictate communication. Emotional trauma, shock, denial and such mental situations prevent the brain from perceiving many things during that time. In such physiological conditions, perception and alertness towards message becomes very low. It also happens during any physical problems like fatigue and illness. Effective communication doesn't take place when the perception and interpretation is selective. When physiological condition of body and mind is not good, people do not want to talk about anything. For example, when a person has lost a close friend in a murder, the person might not want to talk about the incident with the police because of the trauma he/she might be going through.

6.　Physical Condition: Physical condition of body and mind such as pain, disease and sickness changes contents of communication and process used to send any message. Similarly, diseases and infections might affect vital organs needed for communication. Fatigue and stress are also physiological conditions which affect communication flow and act as a barrier. For example, a person having flu is not able to talk for hours like a person without any physiological ailment. Another example is a person with neurological condition of paralysis, in which the person cannot express even a word but can have some physical ways of expression as tears which is not very effective.

Other physical disabilities also interfere with communication; like a problem with the hands does not let a person write and type. Physiological barriers need medical treatments, therapies or corrective aids to help make effective communication.

(B) Physical Barriers:

Disturbances in communication due to external effects are known as physical barriers. It occurs because of wrong choice of medium, excess communication load, complex and lengthy message. It may also be created because of external defects such as faulty working of telephone, loudspeaker, telegram system or internet, excessive noise, poor ventilation, improper seating arrangement, noise and environmental factors as aeration, light etc. and block communication. Physical barrier is the environmental and natural condition that acts as a barrier in communication in sending a message from sender to receiver. Organizational environment or interior workspace design problems, technological problems and noise are some parts of physical barriers. When messages are sent by the sender, physical barriers like doors, walls, distance, etc. do not let the communication become effective. The barriers are less if the proximity of the sender and the receiver is high and lesser technologies are required. Disturbance in hearing due to thunder, telephone call disconnections, problems in television reception, message not being sent in chat, etc. are some examples of physical barriers of communication. A major cause that physical conditions become a barrier is due to distortion. Distortion is the meaning of a message getting lost during the handling process in communication while encoding and decoding.

Different physical barriers are:

1.   Information Overflow: When information becomes more than that can be received at a particular time by the receiver, then communication fails. The receiver does not have the capacity to get all the information and can miss some important points or misinterpret the meaning of the whole message altogether. The message will not get the desired outcome causing the communication to not be effective and act as a barrier. Work overload and information duplication also help to cause physical communication barrier.

2.   Noise: Noise is the disruption found in the environment of the communication. It interrupts the communication process and acts as a barrier as it makes the message less accurate, less productive and unclear. It might even prevent the message from reaching the receiver. There are many kinds of noise in the communication process such as physical noise, written noise, technological noise, etc.

- **Physical noise** is the disturbance that occurs due to outside or background disturbance and environment. This type of noise occurs in mostly all kinds of communication like face to face, written, etc.
- **Written noise** like bad handwriting or typing is also taken as a physical barrier.
- **Technological noise** is the noise that occurs in the medium or channel like no sound while talking on phone or message sending failure in chats.

All of the mentioned types of noises are included as physical communication barriers.

3.   Environment or Climate: Thunder, rain, wind and other environmental factors create noise which cannot be stopped and disturb the message flow. Natural noise is present in the environment which disturbs the communication. Communication is also affected by people being concerned about their own lives which do not let the sender and receiver focus on the message. This is the environment of the particular person. Context (natural environment or person's immediate situation) of the communication also acts and causes to be a barrier as the context might not be right for the particular message to be sent.

4.   Unstable temperature: It makes people unfocused on creating the message. If temperature of a place is too high or low, people cannot concentrate on the information they are sending. It promotes uncomfortable feelings which lead to environmental and physical barrier to communication.

5.   Lack of Aeration and Light: In absence of proper ventilation and light, whether sunlight or electricity, one may not be comfortable and they hamper the free flow of message, thus acting as barriers.

6.   Time and Distance: If a message is not sent in the appropriate time, the message will not have the effect that it should have, as the intention will not be met. This causes barriers in communication. So, the time of the message should be accurate. A person from

Asia will not be able to Skype a person in the U.S. if the time zone difference is wrong and the second person is sleeping. The geographical distance also affects the message. Distance adds more requirements and barriers to communication as greater the distance; the more technical channels are needed. The sender and receiver need to include machines as mediums, encoding, decoding, etc. Face to face communication has the least physical communication barrier and are easier as there as more communication channels.

7.   Medium Disturbance or Technical Problem: Mediums and channels of communication must be decided upon by the role it plays, distance that must be covered, disturbances that might arise, etc. The medium that is suitable for a particular distance with the least noise should be used for communication. If not, then the medium itself acts as a communication barrier and disrupts communication flow. Every kind of medium has one or more defects and disadvantages over another. Mediums have to use network facilities which might lead to technical and technological problems. Mechanical and technical breakdowns such as computer virus or crash or no network coverage can happen anytime. Thus, mediums must not always be trusted to be totally effective.

8.   Workspace Design: If the employees' workspaces are far away from the room of employers, they will not be able to communicate with the employers, take proper orders, make plans, get feedbacks and suggest new ideas. They must work through phones or emails. These mediums have more noise and other technical problems than face to face communication. In this way, workspace designs act as a physical barrier to effective communication. Seating arrangements and physical comfort also fosters or impairs communication. Likewise, organizational structures also act as a barrier to communication. A person has to go through their superior to communicate or to send any message to the main authority of the organization. They cannot talk directly which disturbs the flow of message and alters the meaning of the message. Thus, new concepts like open workspace designs and parallel communication approaches have been emerging to challenge this type of physical communication barrier.

Physical factors obstruct effective communication, in any form of communication. If physical barriers are reduced or eliminated, the communication becomes effective as there is less distortion and interference.

(C) Cultural Barriers:

According to **Joynt** and **Warner**, culture is the pattern of taken-for-granted assumptions about how a given collection of people should think, act, and feel as they go about their daily affairs. Culture is all socially transmitted behaviour, arts, architectures, languages, signs, symbols, ideas, beliefs, norms, traditions, rituals, etc. which is learnt and shared in a particular social group of the same nationality, ethnicity, religion, etc. Culture is handed down from one generation to another. It gives people their way of seeing the world and interpreting life. A single culture has many sub-cultures. Cultural diversity makes communication difficult as the mindset of people of different cultures are different, the language, signs and symbols are also different. Different cultures have different meaning of words, behaviours and gestures. Culture also gives rise to prejudices, ethnocentrism, manners and opinions. It forms the way people think and behave. When people belonging to different cultures communicate, these factors can become barriers.

The way you communicate is affected by the culture you were brought up in. The opposite is also true. Culture is, to a large extent, determined by the way we communicate. In America, people communicate freely and that is a part of their culture. In Germany, an Indian who is used to being very indirect with his communication might find their direct way of speaking rude. Being direct is part of the German culture and it is reflected in the way they communicate. Communication shapes culture and culture shapes communication.

1.   **Language:** There are billions of people in the world who do not understand English or cannot communicate in English properly. Not speaking properly can cause various misunderstandings and be a barrier to communication. Different cultures have developed their own language as a part of their heritage. People are comfortable communicating in their own language whereas have to work hard to learn new languages. Even when people try to express in their own language, many misunderstandings arise. It becomes more profound in people speaking different languages.

2.   **Signs and Symbols (Semantics):** Non-verbal communication cannot be relied upon in communication between people from different cultures as that is also different like language. Signs, symbols and gestures vary in different cultures. For example, the sign "thumbs up" is taken as a sign of approval and wishing luck in most of the cultures but is taken as an insult in Bangladesh. Similarly, the "V" hand gesture with palm faced outside or inside means victory and peace in US, but back of hand facing someone showing the sign is taken as insulting in many cultures. The culture sets some meanings of signs like the ones mentioned above, which might not be the same in another culture.

3.   **Stereotypes and Prejudices:** Stereotyping is the process of creating a picture of a whole culture, over generalizing all people belonging to the same culture as having similar characteristics and categorizing people accordingly. It is a belief about a certain group and is mostly negative. Stereotyping can be done on the basis of many things like nationality, gender, race, religion, ethnicity, age, etc. For example, Asian students are stereotyped to be good at Math which is a positive stereotype. But, there is also cultural stereotype of all people following a particular religion like Islam as being violent and that is negative stereotyping. Negative stereotyping creates prejudices as it provokes judgemental attitudes. People look at those cultures as evil and treat the people following the religion wickedly. Media is a tool of mass communication which promotes stereotypes and prejudices and creates more communication barriers.

4.   **Behaviour and Beliefs:** Cultural differences causes behaviour and personality differences like body language, thinking, communication, manners, norms, etc. which leads to

miscommunication. For example, in some cultures eye contact is important whereas in some it is rude and disrespectful. Culture also sets specific norms which dictates behaviour as they have guidelines for accepted behaviour. It explains what is right and wrong. Every action is influenced by culture like ambitions, careers, interests, values, etc.

Beliefs are also another cause for cultural barriers. For instance, mostly, people who believe in God can cope with their lows of life easily than atheists but atheists are more hard-working at all times which relates to their behaviour and communication. Appropriate amount of emotion that must be displayed is also different in different cultures. Roles are defined by culture. Good communication only occurs between people with different cultures if both accept their differences with an open mind.

5.   Ethnocentrism: Ethnocentrism is the process of dividing cultures as "us" and "them". The people of someone's own culture are categorized as the in-group and the other culture is the out-group. There is always greater preference given to the in-group. There is an illusion of out-group as evil and inferior. This evaluation is mostly negative. If the culture is similar to us, then it is good and if is dissimilar, it is bad. Others' culture is evaluated and assessed with the standard being their own culture. Ethnocentrism affects the understanding of message, and encourages hostility. For example, the books in schools use reference of their own culture to describe other cultures by either showing common things or differences.

6.   Religion: Similar to ethnocentrism and stereotyping, religion also disrupts communication as it creates a specific image of people who follow other religions. People find it difficult to talk to people who follow different religions. Religious views influence how people think about others. It creates differences in opinions. For example, in Pakistan, the Christians have to speak up for their rights as the majority is of Islam and the Christians are discriminated. There is also a lack of communication between these religious groups.

There are other cultural barriers like frames of reference, political opinions, priorities of life, age, etc. Cross cultural communication is not only a barrier but also an opportunity for creativity, new perspectives, and openness to new ideas and unity in the world. To make communication effective, the causes of cultural communication barriers must be eliminated as much as possible. Cross cultural understanding must be increased as it decreases communication barrier caused by culture difference.

(D) Language or Linguistic Barriers:

Language is needed for any kind of communication; even people with speech impairments communicate with sign language and brail. Communication becomes difficult in situations where people don't understand each other's language. The inability to communicate using a language is known as language or linguistic barrier to communication. Language barriers are the most common communication barriers which cause misunderstandings and misinterpretations between people. Most of the people in the world do not speak English or, even if they use, it is their second or third language. If the speaker and receiver do not use the same language and words, there is no meaning to the communication. Not using the words that the other person understands makes communication ineffective and prevents messages from being conveyed. This includes improper encoding/decoding, by-passing, denotations, connotations, using different linguistic codes or even use of non-standard language like using different varieties of language.

1.   Difference in Language: Difference in language is the most obvious barrier to communication as two people speaking two different languages cannot communicate with each other. For example, an American goes to China. The person does not understand Chinese and most people in China do not understand English. So, when the person speaks, the communication is worthless as the other Chinese person doesn't understand it.

2.   Regional Accents, Dialects and Pidgin: The accents and dialect (use of words) of people belonging to different places differs even if their language is same. Though the languages are technically the same in people using different dialects and accents, the meanings, implications and interpretations of words are different, which may lead to various kinds of conflicts. Similarly, pidgin is the simplified language used between people who do not speak common language. The implications of words and phrases can create misunderstandings. For example, the abbreviation "LOL" used in chat language used to mean Lots of Love before, which changed to Laugh Out Loud. If a person says LOL, the second person can interpret the meaning in any way they want or from their understanding. People use both the abbreviations according to the context and need.

3.   Absence of Clear Speech: People who speak in a soft voice cannot be understood. The sender might be saying something whereas the receiver might understand something else. Though speaking a common language, people might have difficulty understanding the meaning of the message and the feedback. This might also be a cause of obstruction in communication.

4.   Use of Jargons and Slang: Jargons are the technical words used in communication. It might be different according to different professions, specialty and technical field of a person. For example, technical words used by doctors and lawyers are extremely different. If they start talking, both of them will not get what the other is talking about. Some jargons like adjournment (jargon used by lawyers and police used for delaying a trial for defendant); BP (medical jargon for blood pressure), etc. are only used by people in similar professions which might be a cause for language barrier. Similarly, the use of slang also makes communication ineffective. For example, the use of word "grass" to describe marijuana can act as a barrier for people who do not know the meaning of the slang usage.

5.   Word Choice: The choice of words used in describing anything must be considered before communicating. The words used by a particular person to show their agreement on something can be taken as sarcasm which is negative in nature. Words with two meanings, homonyms, homographs, homophones should always be avoided as it doesn't send the proper meaning and can be interpreted in any way. So, the message will not be sent as intended which acts as a type of language barrier in communication.

6. **Literacy and Linguistic Ability:** Some people have low vocabulary in a particular language whereas some very high. Though literacy and education increases the need to learn new words, it might not be the only reason. People can increase their vocabulary by reading and with their own interest too. Vocabulary is also less if a person uses the language as their unofficial language. Likewise, linguistic ability is the capability of a person in a particular language. If a person with high vocabulary and linguistic ability talks with another with low ability, the second person will not understand the words used leading to miscommunication of the whole message.

7. **Grammar and Spelling:** Grammar and spelling becomes a barrier in communication as people from different parts of the world can be using it differently even in a particular word. Similarly, grammar and spelling mistakes create a huge communication barrier in written communication. For example, a person makes a mistake of typing 'done' as 'don'. The spelling and grammar checker of the computer does not label it as wrong as 'don' is also a correct word. But, the word can change the whole meaning of the sentence or make the sentence not understandable.

8. **Improper Encoding:** It is a recurrent barrier in the process of communication. Since the message is not encoded correctly proper decoding is not possible and it may lead to confusion and misunderstanding. Messages should be presented in a linguistic code familiar to one's audience. If the audience is not able to follow the language/dialogue/jargon, a communicative failure will definitely occur.

9. **Bypassing:** The term bypassing refers to misunderstanding resulting from missed meanings because of the use of abstract words and phrases on which both sender and receiver do not agree. In order to avoid bypassing you should use familiar words with concrete meaning so that there is no scope for confusion.

10. **Frame of Reference**: Your frame of reference is individual to you as it is based on your experiences, exposure, education, personality and several other arguments. If you analyze everything with your frame of reference then it may again lead to confusion and misunderstanding of the message.

11. **Partial or Marginal Listening**: It can distort the intent of the message. The receiver could be paying heed partially to spoken material and partially to his thought process. In such instances he is sure to misunderstand the intent of the spoken material.

12. **Poor Retention**: Poor retention either on the part of the sender or on the part of the receiver can create problem or may lead to misunderstanding.

13. **Body Language and Gestures:** When what you speak and your body language (kinesics) is different, the listener can get offended. Inconsistent body language creates

conflict. Sarcasm and contrasts make people confused or doubtful about the intentions. Action and language must always go together to make people trust you. For example, if someone requests you with a catapult posture (hands and elbows behind head) which is used to show intimidation, you will interpret the request as an order and might resist doing it.

These are some of the most common causes of language barriers in communication. There are many other causes too like language disabilities, noise, distance or use of metaphors or similes which can be included in other barriers like physiological and physical. Some language barriers can be overcome with practice or other ways like translation, interpreter, language classes, visual methods, etc. whereas some barriers act as problems in a person's whole life. These barriers must not be present to make the communication effective.

(E) Semantic Gap/Semantic Barriers:

The incorrect or careless use of language especially when it is related to words and their meanings is called a semantic barrier. If a person uses a word with multiple meanings, the receiver gets an incorrect message. It is because of the improper pronunciation, incorrect spellings and poor grammar. In language, incorrect pronunciation marks also create a barrier to communication process. Semantics is the study of meaning, signs and symbols used for communication.

The word is derived from "sema", a Greek word meaning signs. Semantic barriers to communication are the symbolic obstacles that distort the sent message in some other way than intended, making the message difficult to understand. The meaning of words, signs and symbols might be different from one person to another and the same word might have hundreds of meanings. So, when a message is sent by a sender to a receiver, it might be interpreted wrongly in a communication process causing misunderstandings between them. This can happen due to different situations that form the semantic of the sender and the receiver, known as the semantic barrier. It also arises due to language, education, culture and place of origin (dialect or accent) or most likely their experiences. It is similar to and related to language barriers in a communication. Different semantic barriers are:

1. **Denotative Words:** Direct meaning of any word which must be shared by two people to understand each other is the denotative meaning. The barriers that arise due to the definition or meaning of a word used differently by sender and receiver are denotative barriers of communication. They disagree on the meaning of a word as they are unaware of the other person's meaning. For example, the meaning of braces, which is used to define the metallic structure to adjust teeth in American English, means a part of clothing in British English.

2. **Connotative Words:** The implied meaning of a word is known as connotative meaning. Connotative barrier in communication refers to the difference of meaning according to different abstract situations, contexts, actions and feelings. Both the

communicators know both meanings of the word, but use only one meaning according to the context, which might be being used differently in the context. For example, the word astonish can be used to describe surprise as well as startle. The words, when used by someone, can have any of the meaning. The context in which it is used will only let the receiver know what the sender means. Another example is the word god, which is used differently by people following different religions.

3.　　**Homophones:** Homophones are words with the same pronunciation but different meanings and might have different spellings too. For example, the words buy, by and bye. They have the same pronunciation, but different meanings and spellings.

4.　　**Homonyms:** Homonyms are words which have the same pronunciation and their spellings are mostly same, but the intended meaning is different. For example, the noun "bear" and the verb "bear" have different meanings but the same pronunciation and spelling.

5.　　**Homographs:** Homographs are words that have the same spelling but the pronunciation and meaning are different. For example, "The research leads to the discovery of lead". In this sentence, both the words have the same spelling, but different pronunciation and different meanings. These words can be interpreted wrongly when used unknowingly causing a semantic barrier in the communication process. This, in turn, makes the communication ineffective.

6.　　**Cultural Difference:** Many words have fixed meanings in different norms. So, confusion arises in communication due to the meaning of different signs and symbols in different cultures, causing a semantic barrier. The use of the "swastika" symbol in Hinduism and in Germany by the Nazi party can be taken as an example. The symbol was used by Hitler for his dictatorship and is taken as something to fear, whereas "swastika" in Hinduism takes it as auspicious and lucky. People belonging to these two cultures interpret the symbol differently and when these people talk or use the symbol, it can lead to conflicts.

7.　　**Difference in Use of Words:** Words can mean something different in two different languages even though the words have the same pronunciation and spelling. People do not know many languages, so the word used in some language might have a different meaning in the language the person understands. The unfamiliarity with the word might make the listener react in a bad way. The receiver might not understand the message or understand it in a way which is not intended. Sequence of use of words must also be taken care of. Technical words or jargons are also understood differently if the receiver does not have proper knowledge. For example, the word "concha" in Spanish means shell whereas it means the female sexual anatomy in an abusive sense in Argentina.

8.　　**Use of Ambiguous Words:** A single word can be used in various ways and they have different meanings. The meaning must be clear of all the words used in every sentence. If the meaning of a particular word can be interpreted in many ways, such a word should not be used unless there are no other alternatives. The words people choose to convey their message makes a communication effective or ineffective. Relative words like bright, love, big, small, good, bad, etc. have their meanings only when compared to or in relation to some other things. For example, "a small fish" can be interpreted as of any size. But if the word is used as "a fish smaller than a marble", then the size can be predicted properly.

Differences in Dialects: People from different parts of the world use different dialects for the same language and pronounce a word differently. People, who speak more than one language, cannot speak a particular language they use less in the same way as the people for whom it is their native language or mother tongue. The mother tongue or the language used most is always prominent and affects the pronunciation of other languages. Dialects or use of different words to give the same meaning according to places makes communication less effective. It causes a semantic barrier as the meaning of the words is different. For example, the style (dialect) of speaking English by an Australian is different from that of an American. People from Australia use the word "autumn" whereas Americans use the word "fall".

(F) Gender Barriers:

Even in a workplace where women and men share equal stature, knowledge and experience, differing communication styles may prevent them from working together effectively. These gender barriers can be inherent or may be related to gender stereotypes and the ways in which men and women are taught to behave as children. Although not all men or all women communicate the same way as the rest of their gender, researchers have identified several traits that tend to be more common in one gender or the other. Understanding these tendencies is the key in creating a work environment that fosters open communication among all employees.

1.   Emotional Vs. Factual: In the "Forbes" article "How to Be a Part of the Male Conversations at Work," author Heather R. Huhman reports that women focus more on feelings and tend to talk about people while men focus more on facts and logic and tend to talk about tangible things such as business or sports. In addition, women use communication to gain insight and understanding, often by asking a lot of questions. Men, on the other hand, communicate primarily to give and get information and are less likely to ask questions.

2.   Motivations: When women meet new people, they focus on learning about the other person and on attempting to earn the other person's trust by showing an interest in him, explains relationship author John Gray. Men, however, focus on establishing their credibility by talking about their achievements, their responsibilities at work and what they have to offer. They expect women to do the same and may not take a woman seriously if she doesn't quickly establish what she can do as a professional.

3.   Misunderstandings: Gender specialist Barbara Annis says many men report that a woman may interpret what they say in a way they didn't expect, causing men to feel unsure about how to approach a topic when discussing it with a woman. When women and men attempt to communicate with no understanding of the other's communication style, they may come across in a way they didn't intend. For example, because women tend to focus more on relationship-building when meeting new people, men may doubt their professionalism. On the other hand, because men tend to be more direct and focused on their achievements, women may perceive them as too aggressive.

4.   Effects of Differences: The differences in the way men and women communicate can lead inadvertently to conflict, inhibiting communication between colleagues and hindering productivity. In her "Forbes" article, Huhman quotes gender diversity expert Connie Glaser, who says, "The problem between men and woman in the workplace is not the fact that they play by a different set of rules. The problem is that they don't know these rules." Huhman adds that when this lack of understanding causes disagreement, men may be able to move on more quickly than women, for whom the conflict has more widespread and long-lasting effects.

(G) Interpersonal Communication:

Many workplaces strive to create strong teamwork to improve productivity and foster a more enjoyable work environment. However, common barriers that get in the way of effective communication can make it more difficult to create a sense of collaboration among the workforce. Communication barriers can take on a variety of forms.

1.   Walls and Doors: Physical barriers such as high cubicle walls and closed office doors can hinder effective communication in the workplace, as they can make workers seem less accessible to each other. To facilitate communication, organizations can create a more open workplace layout that is free of high walls and doors where workers have close proximity to each other while still enjoying personal space. This type of layout can also help to remove the sense that some people have elevated status that can hinder communication between supervisors and their subordinates.

2.   Cultural and Language Differences: In multicultural workplaces, cultural and language differences can impede communication. Cultural barriers can also take the form of a unique workplace environment where workers are expected to behave in a particular way to gain acceptance. For example, some workplaces exhibit an autocratic culture where differing points of view are not tolerated, which can limit communication. In addition, language barriers can result not only when workers have different native languages but when they use jargon, buzzwords or terminology that is unfamiliar to new workers, who may feel excluded until they can master the lexicon.

3.   Gender Issues: Differences between genders can create communication barriers in a number of ways. For instance, in a traditionally male-dominated work environment, women may have difficulty getting their ideas accepted, or they may be treated harshly or even ignored. Different communication styles can result in barriers, as men and women do not always form and express thoughts in the same manner. Some men may feel uncomfortable with or even resent working for a female supervisor, which can also get in the way of effective communication.

4.   Competition: In a highly competitive work environment, workers may be more concerned with their own career advancement than helping or communicating effectively with their co-workers. An atmosphere of distrust can also result, making it difficult for workers to perform in a collaborative manner due to fear of "backstabbing." As a result, workers may be reluctant to share important information with one another. Competition can also result in power struggles, where certain individuals or factions within an organization fail to communicate with each other.

(H) Intrapersonal Communication:

Personal factors like difference in judgment, social status, social value, inferiority complex, attitude, pressure of time, inability to communicate etc. widen the psychological distance between the sender and receiver. Credibility gap, that is, inconsistency between what one says and what one does, can also act as a barrier to communication. It may also be because of the faulty sensory organs, improper hearing ability, poor health, weakness, poor state of mind etc. Personal barriers are real or imagined hindrances between you and the success you want to achieve. The key to overcoming personal barriers is to identify what keeps you from reaching your goals, and then take steps to remove those impediments. While the process may sound simple, overcoming personal barriers can be one of the hardest things you have every accomplished.

"Intrapersonal" means happening within the individual's mind or self; "interpersonal" means happening with others, interactions between the individual and outside others. It's a negative voice that keeps us down-spirited, downtrodden, and can cause us to stop trying. These thoughts are actually a form of self-protection, to keep us from getting emotionally hurt. But when the inner rant is out of control, this help does more harm than good. When this is the case, you need to take back the control and shut down the negative inner voice, which is the biggest impediment to intrapersonal communication. There are many of those, such as –

1.   Fear: Fear of failure is one of the hardest barriers to overcome, but just as debilitating are fear of success and fear of change. Whatever fear is keeping you from reaching your goals becomes a barrier that prevents you from being the best person you can be. Once you determine what you are afraid of, visualize the worst thing that can happen; then, visualize the best thing. Often, the return for facing the fear and overcoming it is better than anything that would happen to you if you fail.

2.   Time: Everyone has the same 24 hours in a day and the same number of days in a year. How time is used can be a barrier for one person and an asset to another. When you find yourself using a lack of time as an excuse repeatedly, odds are that you have time management problems. Take a look at what you do with the time you have and determine if you are making the best use of your time. Does what you are doing with your time actually make you happy or does it feel as if you are doing filler projects until something better comes along? You may be surprised how many minutes you waste in your day that could be used to better purposes.

3.   Energy: The intrapersonal barrier of a lack of energy is a strange conundrum, especially when it comes to exercising, weight loss and health problems. Lack of exercise, being overweight and health problems, such as depression will make you feel tired. However, exercising, losing weight and engaging in activities are often the very solutions to low energy. When you face this problem, take baby steps toward overcoming a low energy level. For example, instead of exercising 30 minutes at a time, break your exercise regimen into short spurts several times a day. Eventually, you will have more energy to take on more exercise at one time.

4.   Resources: When a lack of family support, money, education or experience prevents you from doing something you really want to do, you may feel thwarted before you have ever begun reaching your goal. Look for alternate resources.

5.   Attitude: Having a closed mind, being judgmental, stereotyping are all barriers to communication. When you think you know already and are not willing to be open-minded then no communication can cross that mental barrier.

6.   Not Listening: We hear but we don't necessarily listen. The best definition of true listening is to be willing to be changed by what you hear. Not listening because we think we already know what the person is going to say, or because our ego can't allow looking stupid or being wrong, or because we're too distracted to give the other person our full attention – is a barrier to communication.

7.   High Emotions: When anyone is in a highly charged emotional state, elated, depressed, grieving, raging mad – the emotion is a big barrier to communication. It's nearly impossible to control the emotion to think and communicate clearly until it has run its course and rational thinking returns.

(I) Psychological Barriers:

These barriers depend on the mentality and personality of the human being. They may be because of depression, emotions, wrong timings of message, complexes, defective communication network, language differences, wrong pronunciation, and improper vocabulary, receiver's attention, sender's or receiver's background etc. These develop a negative thinking or misunderstanding. Barriers may also arise due to emotional attitude because when emotions are strong, it is difficult to know the frame of mind of the person or group and emotional attitude of   sender and receiver after transmission and understanding of message. A barrier is any obstacle that prevents us from reaching our goal. Any hindrance to communication stops the intended meaning of our message from reaching our audience. Some of these barriers are obvious, for example, a physical disability like deafness, while some are more subtle and difficult to pinpoint. Psychological barriers belong to the latter group and can seem impossible to overcome unless we understand their underlying causes. The psychological barrier of communication is the influence of psychological state of the communicators (sender and receiver) which creates an obstacle for effective communication. Communication is highly influenced by the mental condition that the communicators are in and is disturbed by mental disturbance. If the people involved in communication are not emotionally well, they won't be able to communicate properly. Every person's mind is unique and communication does not work like that in machines or in numbers. The people who are involved in the communication matter as much as the message. For example, if your boss doesn't trust you, he/she will only send selective information, which makes the communication ineffective.

1.   **Lack of Attention:** When a person's mind is distracted or preoccupied with other things, the person is not able to form a proper message, listen to what others tell him/her, interpret the message as required and give proper feedback. The communication will face problems and becomes ineffective. A person in mourning, for instance, does not want to listen to other people giving advice. A person might be preoccupied by the problems of his/her professional life or personal life, which affects both.

2.   **Poor Retention:** Retention of information is the capacity of the memory of the brain to store information and the way the brain stores information in the memory. The brain does not store all the information it comes across, but only the ones it deems useful for future. So, half the information is lost in the retention process. Similarly, the brain also loses information that is old and not taken as useful with time. Extracting the information is also a process in the formation of the message. Here, the brain tries to remember the required information, the fragments of which have already been lost. For example, you were told about a friend coming to meet you before a month and had been given the person's name, address, phone number, etc. Now, you have to communicate the information to somebody else. At the time, you only remember the name and address and forget the phone number. The truth can change or distort due to poor retention which acts as barrier to communication.

3.   **Distrust and Defensiveness:** Communication is successful when the communicators trust each other. Lack of trust makes them derive negative meaning of the message and they ignore the message. When a person tries to force his/her own ideas and opinions, then the receiver does not listen. If the receiver does not agree to the message provided or thinks of it as a threat, he/she will not listen to it. Similarly, when the message is not transferred across to the receiver, the communication fails. For example, I don't trust a friend; I will only give the details, of what is happening in my personal life which I think are harmless.

4.   **Perceptions, Viewpoints, Attitudes and Opinions:** Perception is the mindset using which people judge, understand and interpret everything. Each person has his/her own perception of reality which is shaped from mental and sensory experiences. Likewise, viewpoint is also a mindset to look at the world. The sender might have a particular viewpoint that is not shared by the receiver. The sender does not explain the viewpoint but

takes the viewpoint as granted. The message is not understood by the receiver as must have been understood, creating a barrier to effective communication. Attitude is the established way in which we think and feel about things and ideas which also creates a psychological communication barrier. For example, a person takes females to be weak which is the person's perception. He/she tells that to someone who does not think so. This causes a misunderstanding between the two. Everything they communicate after that becomes unsuccessful as the views of those persons is already set.

5.   Emotions: Anyone who isn't in a good mood is likely to talk less or talk negatively. A preoccupied mind is not good at communicating. For example, when a person is angry, he/she might say things they regret later. Even when listening to someone else talk an angry person might easily misinterpret the message. Various other emotions like fear, nervousness, confusion, mistrust and jealousy affect communication process. For example, a person having extreme moods of happiness will laugh at anything at all said to him/her. The same person when sad will cry or get angry at insignificant situations.

6.   Closed Mind and Filtering: Man is selfish by nature and puts his own needs and problems above all else. This sometimes leads people to filter information that someone is trying to convey to them. This might be due to mistrust, competition, jealousy, or the view that the message is insignificant. For example, a senior in a company does not want the junior to do better at work and so the person filters the information and does not provide crucial information that could help the junior. The junior therefore will not be able to complete the work properly and progress in ranks. Similarly, when a person is close-minded, the person will have fixed opinions on many things which the person believes resolutely. The person will interpret any information in a negative way.

7.   Premature Evaluation: Some people are always in a hurry by habit. These kinds of people most likely make quick judgements and jump into conclusions. They do not consider all aspects of the information such as social, cultural, economic, etc. and often end up taking quick and wrong decisions. It is important to hear the whole message to make proper judgments because they can't be changed easily once made. For example, a person in a hurry talks on the phone; the person does not listen to half the message and takes a decision which is wrong in the situation.

8.   Rigidity: Rigidity in a communication means the meaning attached to various words and expressions varies from person to person. Some people hold certain views on various matters that they hardly listen to the other person in view of their rigid stand on matters. This leads to ineffective communication.

9.   Extreme Opinion: People with extreme opinions behave in such a way that if a person is good in one area they consider him good in every aspect of life. This happens in the other way too. This leads to ineffective communication.

Psychological barriers affect communication more as information is formed in the brain and is sent by people with various psychological conditions which differ from one moment to another. Information is as effective as the people involved in making it.

(I) Emotional Barriers:

Whether you want to run a successful business or maintain close ties to friends, family and love interests, effective communication is one important element to keep in mind. Effective communications involves more than just speaking; it involves active listening as well. However, strong negative emotions can interfere with one or both of these aspects of communication. This can lead to miscommunication, hurt feelings and even severed ties. Learn about common emotional roadblocks to communication, so you can find ways to clear your mind before engaging others.

1.　Anger: Whether a heated argument has you upset with the person you're speaking to or a bad day has you on edge with everyone around you, anger can cause you to lash out and say things you don't mean. Anger can also affect the way your brain processes information given to you. For example, angry people have difficulty processing logical statements, limiting their ability to accept explanations and solutions offered by others, says John Schafer, a former behavioural analyst for the FBI, in his Psychology Today article, "Controlling Angry People." With this in mind, remove yourself from communication until you feel you can collect your thoughts, think clearly and hold back potentially hurtful and undue comments.

2.　Pride: Pride hinders listening. Pride or the need to be right all the time will not only annoy others, it can shut down effective communication. For example, you might focus only on your perspective, or you might come up with ways to shoot down other people before you even listen to their points. The drive to win every argument or get the last word often spawns from overcompensation, or trying to cover emotional insecurities with a sense of superiority, suggests other people might find you easier to communicate with when you accept your imperfections from time to time.

3.　Depression: Depression, whether clinical or short-term, can cause a person to isolate himself and block out communication, altogether. Depression can also lead to cold feelings toward loved ones, or irritating and sarcastic remarks, suggests the University of Florida's Counselling and Wellness Center in an article titled, "How to Deal with Depression." However, those who are depressed are often the ones in most need of social support. While short-term sadness will eventually pass—and perhaps more quickly if you open yourself to communication—clinical depression might require the assistance of a mental health expert.

4.　Anxiousness: Anxiety has a negative impact on the part of your brain that manages creativity and communication skills, explains the University of Michigan's Department of Psychiatry in "Anxiety." For example, your constant worries can hinder your ability to concentrate on the information you are giving or receiving. Irritability and restlessness might also push others away from you, decreasing the chances of effective or lengthy communication. While a mental health professional should address anxiety disorders such as post-traumatic stress disorder or phobias— typical anxiety, like the anxiety you feel before giving a speech—can be managed with relaxation exercises.

(K) Organizational Barriers:

The organizational barriers refer to the hindrances in the flow of information among the employees that might result in a commercial failure of an organization. The major organizational barriers are listed below.

1.　**Organizational Rules and Policies:** Often, organizations have the rule with respect to what message, medium, and mode of communication should be selected and due to the stringent rules, the employees hesitate sending any message. Similarly, the organizational policy defines the relationship between the employees and the way they shall communicate with each other maintaining their levels of position in the organization. Such as, if the company policy is that all the communication should be done in writing, then even for a small message the medium used should be written. This leads to delay in the transmission of the message and hence the decision- making gets delayed.

2.　**Status or Hierarchical Positions in the Organization:** In every organization, the employees are divided into several categories on the basis of their levels of the organization. The people occupying the upper echelons of the hierarchy are superior to the ones occupying the lower levels, and thus, the communication among them would be formal. This formal communication may often act as a barrier to effective communication, such as the lower level employee might be reluctant in sending a message to his superior because of a fear in his mind of sending a faulty or wrong message. Subordinates tend to convey only those things which the superiors will appreciate. This creates distortion in upward communication.

3.　**Organizational Facilities:** Organizational facilities mean the telephone, stationery, translator, etc., which are being provided to employees to facilitate communication. When these facilities are adequately offered to the employees, the communication tends to be timely, accurate and according to the need. In the absence of such facilities, the communication may get adversely affected.

4.　**Filtering by Senders and Selective Perception by Receivers:** Prejudices of people make them only listen to and interpret the things they want to. They always do it their way. They understand the way they want to. Similarly, the senders also send only the information they want to. They withhold the information that they do not want the receiver to understand. Both of them use the words that serve their interests and objectives. The sender filters before sending and the receiver perceives selectively which shapes the meaning of the message. The message must be according to the level of understanding of the receiver and in the same way filtering before sending must be done. For example, a magazine which has middle aged women as target will filter their articles and will not include anything about business. That is filtering. A reader looking at the magazine will skip the articles which is not of his/her interest. That is selective perception.

5.   Complex Organizational Structure: Communication gets affected if there are a greater number of management levels in the organization. With more levels, communication gets delayed and might change before reaching the intended receiver.

Thus, communication is the key factor in the success of any firm, and the communication is said to be effective when the employees interact with each other in such a way that it results in the overall improvement of the self as well as the organization.

Suitable Measures to Overcome Communication Barriers:

The barriers to communication cannot be totally removed; we can try to minimize them up to a great extent because they are an inseparable part of communication. If communication takes place, some or other barriers can also be noticed there. By following some measures these barriers can be controlled or minimized. Following are some of the measures to overcome the barriers to the communication process –

- The proper medium of communication should be used.
- External barriers of faulty channels should be removed and checked frequently.
- Message should be in a simple and clear language.
- For effective communication, personal interaction, proper training should be provided to the authorities.
- Semantic barriers can be overcomed by studying the language carefully. Clear and concise words, proper punctuation marks, correct grammar and correct spellings should be used. Workshops, seminars which create healthy mental atmosphere must be created.

By following the above mentioned measures, the barriers can be overcome up to a great extent if not totally.

2.3 HOW TO MAKE THE COMMUNICATION EFFECTIVE

By learning to communicate effectively our confidence in gaining success in interaction increases. Lack of communication skills often result in depression, shyness, stress, negativity, loneliness etc. On the other hand the ability to communicate well not only sustains relationships but also promotes effectiveness in the job. Organizations look for those employees who can communicate effectively and assertively.

The following points may help in making our communication effective –

- **Self Awareness:** Understanding your personal style of communication will help you to create the desired effect on others. If you are aware of the fact how others perceive you, you may adapt to their styles of communicating. This way you can create a comfortable, congenial environment.
- **Express Yourself Clearly:** Sometimes the way you say something may not mean what you intend to say. Organize thoughts in your mind. This will give proper shape to your expressions and your listeners would understand you better.

- **Active Listener:** Active listening means that you are paying attention to what others say – you are listening with a purpose. Active listening helps you to gain information, obtain directions, understand others, and look at the things from the sender's point of view. It's not easy to concentrate on what someone is saying since only a part of our mind pays attention. Our mind is constantly thinking about other things while listening to someone. To control from drifting, try to repeat the words of the sender in your mind. This helps in concentration. And do not indulge yourself in other activities.

- **Be Positive:** Positive communication is always encouraging. It can be hard to see the positive in everything, but if you try to find positivity, you will definitely find it out. If you go into a conversation with a negative or a defensive tone, your message may not get the desired result. Positive attitude must be applied to listening as well. Do not take positive things for granted or negative as personal offence.

- **Be Honest:** If you do not know something, never hesitate to say no. People can identify with a communicator who admits he is wrong. It will give you credibility in future communication.

- **Be Humble:** The fact that people may be better at doing something should always be kept in mind. Offering some level of humanity will make the environment congenial, encouraging the smooth flow of communication.

- **Use Non-Verbal Communication Effectively:** A great deal of communication is non-verbal like facial expressions, tone of voice, motions, gestures, smiles, posture, eye-contact etc. It may also include the way we wear our clothes. Be sensitive to non-verbal messages. Co-operation in an organization improves if we recognize and respond appropriately to non-verbal cues.

- **Speak Directly and Assertively:** Speak for a purpose and the body language should correspond with your words. Too much communication can be counter-productive. Communicate in the clearest possible way.

- **Avoid Pre-determined Notions:** Being receptive always makes communication easier and effective. Be open to every suggestion and every criticism. Never frame in your mind the pre-determined idea about the people you are communicating with. This may make you prejudiced and the flow of communication may get disturbed.

- **Feedback:** Effective feedback is always specific and not general. Feedback should not contain advice. Constructive feedback is not criticism. Feedback should always be directed to the action and not the person.

Keeping all these points in mind effectiveness of communication can be improved.

EXERCISE

1. What are the barriers to communication?

2. Explain in detail the socio-psychological barriers to communication.

3. How do the following factors affect communication process in an organization?

   (a) Noise, (b) Distance, (c) Status consciousness, (d) Rigid hierarchy, (e) Meetings (f) Abstracting, (g) Slanting, (h) Inferring.

4. Define different comprehensions of reality and how does it function as a barrier to communication.

5. What is effective communication? How could you make your communication effective?

6. Identify the common barriers and describe ways to remove them.

7. Define different comprehensions of reality and how they function as a barrier to communication.

8. How can various barriers be overcome in an organization?

9. What are the inter and intra personal barriers? Explain them.

10. Define organizational barriers.

11. What do you understand by failure of communication?

12. What is meant by miscommunication? Explain.

13. How does miscommunication arise?

14. Write a detailed note on the semantic and psychological barriers of communication.

15. Write short notes on the following –

    (a) Organizational barriers, (b) Semantic barriers, (c) Personal barriers, (d) Psychological barriers.

16. Enumerate the physical barriers to effective communication.

17. How does personal opinions and prejudices of individuals act as barriers to communication?

18. What do you understand by status? How does it hinder the smooth flow of communication?

19. "There can never be perfect communication". Comment giving reasons.

Chapter ... 3

PERSPECTIVES IN COMMUNICATION

◆ LEARNING OBJECTIVES ◆

Objectives of this chapter are:

- *To make the students learn about different perspectives of communication like visual perseption, language, past experiences, prejudices, feelings and environment*
- *To know how to make profitable use of one's past experiences to deal with person in different circumstances.*

3.1 INTRODUCTION

Every discipline offers a unique perspective that we can use to understand human phenomena such as groups, organizations, communities, cultures, and societies. For instance, an *economic perspective* focuses attention on explaining how economies work and how people make decisions about resources and a *psychological perspective* explains the behavior of individuals and groups using ideas related to the cognition, perception, and emotions. A communication perspective not only examines the way that messages transmit information and influence individual and collective behavior; it also examines the way that messages create, sustain, and change cultures and communities. Communication scholars explore the form, content, medium and patterns of messages and how they influence the way that people make meaning and take action. We examine how messages are produced, how they are circulated among a group of people, and how they are interpreted with an eye on the important consequences of messages.

A communication perspective helps us engage some of the most pressing social, political, and cultural issues facing our nation and our world. A communication perspective focuses on the way in which our shared meanings and practices are constituted through language and symbol, the construction of messages, and their dissemination through media, organizations, and society. Despite the old saying, "Sticks and stones may break my bones, but words will never harm me," in fact any message potentially has significant consequences for the way we understand ourselves and our place in the world around us. Communication always makes a difference. To acquire a communication, perspective is thus to learn how to make a positive difference in the world using language, symbols, and messages.

In psychology and the cognitive sciences, sensation is the process of converting of energy from the environment into neural energy. Sensation is the process which our sense organs receive stimulus from the environment, whereas perception is the process of acquiring, interpreting, selecting, and organizing sensory stimulus. That is, perception is the process which an individual selects stimuli, organizes information about those stimuli, and interprets the information. Perceptions are affected by all the events in your life. The past has a tremendous impact on what people perceive. Every single person has a unique perception. People's thinking depends on those experiences as well. So perception is always experiential. A person who has experienced being bitten by a dog would always think that dogs are fear. Whenever he sees a dog, he would show his fear. While one who has not experienced being bitten by a dog would not have this perception.

Perception is the process of making sense out of an experience as well as the imputing of meaning to experience. Our past experiences play a vital role in perception. Learning from previous experiences has a critical effect throughout all the stages of the perceptual process. It will affect the stimulus perceived in the first instance, and then the ways in which that stimulus is understood and processed and finally respond. People respond to those stimuli because of former experiences and, pick out what will be perceived.

Do you remember the first time you met your best friend? What was your initial thought about that person? Did you think they looked scary, funny, smart, stupid or intimidating? Your initial thoughts that ran through your mind were your perceptions of the person. Perception is the processing, interpreting, selecting and organizing of information. Perception's effect on the communication process is all about how the same message can be interpreted differently by different people. In order to communicate effectively, business people need to spend time to fully investigate job applicants. They should also not judge an individual by just first their impression. Perhaps you thought your future best friend was a serious, shy person due to the fact that they dressed conservatively and wore glasses. In the end, your perception could have been incorrect, as your friend turned out to be very extroverted. People can filter out certain information to make it align with their own thoughts, beliefs and judgments.

3.2 VISUAL PERCEPTION

Visual perception is the process of using vision to acquire information about the surrounding environment or situation. Visual perception is the ability to see, organize, and interpret one's environment.

A

For example, your eyes 'took in' the lines as well as the points on the ends of the lines. At the same time, your brain was organizing and making sense of the image. This is a very important process because it gives us the ability to learn new information. Without visual perception, you would not be able to make sense of words that you read, visually recognize common objects, or have the eye-hand coordination required for many daily tasks.

The process of talking in one's environment is referred to as perception. If perception is inaccurate, incorrect or altered in any way – problem with reading, spelling, handwriting, math and comprehension occur. Visual perceptual skills involve the ability to organize and interpret the information that is seen and give it meaning. The importance of visual perceptual skills in academic success is agreed upon by many, acknowledging reading would not be possible without adequate visual perception.

Visual perceptual processing impacts the ability to learn: Without accurate perceptual processing, a student would have difficulty in learning to read, give or follow directions, copy from the whiteboard, visualize objects or past experiences, have good eye-hand coordination, integrate visual information with other senses to do things like ride a bike, play catch, shoot basketball or hear a sound and visualize where it is coming from (like a siren on a police car or ambulance).

Ways of Interpreting Information: Visual perception occurs in two ways. One way is called top-down processing. This theory of perception says that we use our own knowledge and expectations to influence what we see. We draw on our whole understanding of a concept in order to make sense of the individual components.

THE CHT

For example, in the image above, you probably read that as 'the cat'. On closer inspection, the second word is not really a word at all. It says 'CHT'. Because our brains have an expectation of what we will read, we skipped right over the fact that it said CHT instead of CAT. The top-down model of processing explains why we are able to quickly look at new information and understand it. We use our previous experiences to influence learning of new information. For instance, this would explain why we know what a bus is, whether it is a school bus, a public transportation bus, or a double-decker bus. We know what the concept of bus is, so when we see a new color or kind of bus, we can understand that it's still a bus.

The human eye-brain system is arguably the most sophisticated computing system which we have access to. It can easily handle complex visual processing and pattern recognition tasks which would be impossible to attempt on even the most powerful computer. In communication we undertake so many tasks. The task which our visual system excels at is those which were useful to our hunter-gatherer forbears. These tasks include recognizing signs and shapes, discerning colors, judging size and distances, and tracing and extrapolating motion in three dimensions. Most of the times our eyes give us a good sense of the way things are. We can recognize everything, whether it's a face or words and signs written on a page. Sometimes, however, we can be quite misled into seeing effects which are not really present. Images which produce this kind of phenomenon are called visual illusions. They are of many kinds like perspective illusion, geometric illusion, Ponzo illusion, Muller Lyer illusion, Zollnier illusion, horizontal-vertical illusion, color illusion etc.

Visual perceptual skills include several key component areas:

- **Visual Discrimination:** The ability to notice detail differences such as shape, size, color or other dimensional aspects.
- **Form Consistency/Discrimination:** The ability to perceive positional aspect differences and recognize objects when they are in a different orientation or format.
- **Figure Ground or Foreground – Background Differentiation:** The ability to focus on a selected target and screen out or ignore irrelevant images.
- **Spatial Relations:** The ability to recognize the positioning of objects in space.
- **Visual Closure:** The ability to recognize an object, letter or number without seeing the entire object.
- **Visual Sequencing:** The ability to see objects in a particular sequential order.
- **Visual Memory:** The ability to remember forms (letters) and sequences of forms (words) and recognize them quickly when seen again.

When visual information is perceived or processed incorrectly, it cannot be matched or integrated with our other senses. Instead of reinforcing learning experiences, it distracts and interferes. If what is seen cannot be 'trusted', it hinders the ability to learn. Poor visual perceptual processing is not something a student 'outgrows'. If undiagnosed or left untreated, the student with poor visual perceptual processing will continue to fall behind in class even though it may appear they are working harder than other students in the same class.

Paying attention, categorization, memorization and acquisition of knowledge are all cognitive processes. Cognitive processes are cognitive activities that affect our mental content. Visual perception is vital in cognitive processing. Visual perception is the process of absorbing what one sees, organizing it in the brain and making sense of it. One of the most common examples of visual perception's importance in cognitive processes is reading. Looking at the words of a book and being able to make sense of the plot is visual perception at work. Difficulty in visual perception can cause problems with cognitive processes.

Attention, learning, perception, memory and discrimination are all cognitive processes and are aided by visual perception. What is one of the first things that children must master when they begin school? Paying attention! Attention is a cognitive process. Being able to focus and pay attention is the foundation of learning, as one must focus on the subject...for example, the ABCs...in order to retain it. The visual perception skill of visual attention is what allows us to cut out distractions in the environment in order to focus on what is important. For example, a child with poor visual perception might not be able to focus on the teacher if there is a colorful bulletin board and ticking clock also within eyesight.

Learning, or acquisition of knowledge, is a cognitive process that becomes more difficult with poor visual perception. We know that deficits in visual perception can make it difficult to make sense of what one reads. Deficits in visual perception can also make it hard to tell the difference between foreground and background – also known as figure ground skills in visual perception –like seeing white letters in a chalkboard in school or distinguishing between the black letters on white background on a page in a book. Considering that reading is one of the main ways that we acquire knowledge, it is evident how important visual processing is, to learning.

Perception is how we draw conclusions from sensory experiences. Two people may perceive the same sensory experience differently. Imagine two people walk into a restaurant and one person smells pumpkin pie while the other smells fresh baked biscuits. It turns out they are both right as the chef is cooking a thanksgiving feast. Our perception of things can be altered by our interest, past experiences, personality and personal characteristics.

Discrimination is the ability to differentiate between two partially similar objects or two different objects or letters .Visual perception refers to information that is perceived through eyes. Although most children develop the ability to focus visually and to make fine discriminations in visual images as they grow. Good visual perception is an important skill. Children need good visual perception to discriminate well, copy text accurately, develop visual memory of things observed, develop good eye-hand coordination and integrate visual information while using other senses in order to perform tasks like recognizing the source of a sound etc. Visual perception includes color perception and color constancy, shape perception and shape constancy, spatial relations, visual analysis and synthesis, visual conceptualizing, visual discrimination and visual figure – ground distinction.

3.3 LANGUAGE

The primary function of any language is to convey information or to express emotions. But language is also used to maintain social relationships and to identify with a certain section of society. This means that all human languages have two sides: an internal structure concerned with the organization of linguistic information necessary for communication and an external aspect where the manner in which language is expressed carries social significance. A communication perspective focuses on the way in which our shared meanings and practices are constituted through language and symbol, the construction of messages, and their dissemination through media, organization and society.

The different perspectives we experience can be with language as well. How many times have you received an email that seemed to have a certain 'tone to it,' and that perception of tone colored the way that you might have responded? The same words can have very different meanings depending on how we interpret them. Here's another example. What is the meaning of the following phrase?

A woman, without her man is nothing.

Sounds pretty bad at first glance, don't it? Look again. If you add punctuation or change the word emphasis, how does the meaning change?

A woman without her man, is nothing.

The words were the same in both cases. But the meaning has now changed completely. So although we think our meaning may be clear when we use specific words in a certain order, we can't always be certain that the other person will read or hear them in that way.

3.4 OTHER FACTORS AFFECTING PERSPECTIVE

1. Past Experiences:

Imagine that you are in a meeting where you will be discussing changes in your personnel policies at work. What will you bring to that conversation? You might have examples of other company's personnel policies. You might have examples from your own time in the company that demonstrates why you feel that certain changes might need to be made. Or you might come to the table empty-handed, with just a pad of paper and a pen in order to take notes. What influences you to do any of these things? Your past experience. You would bring outside information because you have learned in the past that comparing situations can be helpful in decision-making. You bring examples of your own experience because you have learned in the past that examples can be powerful ways to make your case. Or you come to the table empty-handed because in the past you have felt that your input wasn't valued or you have no past experience in this topic and so you are a 'clean slate' information-wise. In every one of these situations, your communication is being affected by your past experience. You enter a situation, a meeting, or a conversation, with certain expectations of what will happen in that scenario, and you behave accordingly.

Of course, sometimes you want your past experience to influence your future communications. For example, when your team responded positively to the sales tactics you put in place, those same or similar tactics can certainly be successful again but when our negative past experiences stifle our communication or alter our full potential for communicating that we need to be aware.

Past experiences often combine one or a few senses, and are closely associated with our everyday life. Past experience with positive or negative reinforcement in similar situations may have generated strong biases which influence current perceptions. The past experience of the person can greatly affect our perception. Like a situation that is relatable for everyone is waking up in the morning. If you look at the idea of perception, the process of waking up is an interesting one as it determines one's emotions and therefore actions for the rest of the day. For example if you wake up happy in the morning, you are more likely to have an increased level of patience compared to if you wake up on the wrong side of the bed. The knowledge question we extracted from this real life situation stated "To what extent do past experiences affect our perception?" This is related to our real life situation since waking up (past experience) affects how we see situations that day. To further explain this idea, we shared personal experiences, one involving in an un-experienced scuba diver's experience in comparison to his/her instructor. We concluded that although past experiences drastically effects how we perceive situations, it is not the only contributing factor. Another factor is education, for example if the un-experienced scuba diver was already educated, through the studying of books about the ocean, their perception would have been more similar to the one of their instructor.

2. Prejudices:

We all have prejudices. They occur when we take our past experiences with a person and assume that the same type of experience will happen with all people who are similar to the first. Prejudices are partly due to culture and partly due to personal preference or experience. Not all prejudices involve a negative characteristic either; for example, you could consider all of one group to be smart. The problem with prejudices is when they start to influence how or to whom we communicate.

To get an idea of how this could be happening in your workplace, consider how you might complete the phrases below. If you can't think of a way to complete it from your own experience, complete each phrase with a stereotype that you might have heard in the past:

- Women in the workplace are....
- Young people in the workplace are...
- Seniors in the workplace are...
- Working mothers in the workplace are...
- Supervisors at work are...
- The lowest job level workers are...
- Blacks, whites, or (fill in a race) in the workplace are...
- Disabled people in the workplace are...

Prejudices occur when we take an isolated experience with one 'type' of person and then act as if all encounters in the future with people of the same 'type' or with the same characteristics will result in the same experience. When we categorize people like this, we eliminate their individuality. If you are communicating to a person through a perceived prejudice or stereotype, at the very least you are greatly limiting the chances of your communication being successful or producing the desired result. At the most, you are alienating or insulting someone with whom you are trying to build a working relationship. Your goal should be to see each person as an individual that is separate from any preconceived notions you might have about them. It takes practice, but wouldn't you like to be seen and communicated with as an individual and not as a sum of different labels that can be placed on you?

3. Consequences of Prejudice

Like the wide variety of prejudices that exist in societies around the world, the consequences of the prejudices and the behavior influenced by them are similarly varied. Prejudice affects the everyday lives of millions of people across the globe. Prejudice held by individuals unnaturally forces on others who are targets of their prejudice a false social status that strongly influences who they are, what they think, and even the actions they take. Prejudice shapes what the targets of prejudice think about the world and life in general, about the people around them, and how they feel about themselves. Importantly, prejudice greatly influences what people expect from the future and how they feel about their chances for self-improvement, referred to as their life chances. All of these considerations define their very identity as individuals. People acting out their prejudices cause domestic violence, crime, death, and the loss of billions of dollars in lost productivity, property loss, and expense to society, such as cost of court trials and social services provided to victims including psychological counselling, in dealing with dysfunctional (abnormal behaviour) elements of society. Other prejudicial behaviour, such as male teachers favoring calling on male students in a classroom, may be more subtle (less obvious). But its effect can be just as broad-sweeping as the more violent consequences of prejudice. Opportunities in life are lost and personal relationships damaged when people act upon their prejudice. When not acknowledged and confronted, prejudice negatively impacts the lives not only of the victims, but of those holding the prejudice. Prejudice can impose very dramatic or invisible barriers on the individual. Prejudice may result in stigma, a feeling of shame or of lesser social value than others.

Everyday Prejudices: Since multiple prejudices are present throughout society in a complex way, at minimum, the consequences of prejudice are always presented in subtle, if not more obvious, ways. For example, because people are largely aware of the prejudices held by others toward them, the prejudice has a self-fulfilling effect. This means people behave the way others expect them to behave. Similarly, people holding a prejudice treat others differently based on how the person with prejudices expects the others to behave or how the person with prejudices wants the others to behave. These behavioral expectations are often based on stereotypes. Stereotypes are an oversimplified prejudgment of others using physical or behavioral characteristics, usually exaggerated, that supposedly apply to every member of that group. In addition, people behave differently from person to person when interacting with others, depending on whether they expect hostility from others either in attitude or in action. Studies have shown that a person targeted by stereotype expectations held by others may end up behaving as the stereotype. More generally, a person is likely to behave as the other person expects him to behave. All of these behaviors mean that prejudice, or anticipated prejudices, affect everyday interactions with almost everyone a person comes in contact with.

Consequences of everyday prejudice go beyond simply shaping relationships between people. People are relentlessly assaulted by value judgements based on skin colour, social class, gender, religious affiliation, political views, and so on. Such constant exposure to ridicule and discrimination leads to a lowered self-esteem. Those subjected to such prejudice become unsure where they belong in society. They develop hatred and anger directed both outwardly at those holding prejudices against them and inwardly for having the supposed traits that attract such prejudices. Such prejudices are destructive of individuals and society. But they extract a hidden cost as well by prohibiting individuals from living up to their true potential. Very small but harmful prejudicial actions can create barriers for entire populations, such as women, seeking to enjoy the benefits of participating in mainstream society. Often these actions are unintentional, caused by prejudices a person is little aware he has. However, many times they are intentional acts meant to degrade another person considered inferior. It is sometimes difficult to determine if an act is unintended and simply insensitive or meant as intentional hostility. Regardless of intentions, the consequence of action is often the same. Many times the person who is the target of such prejudicial actions is placed in difficult situations. Any protest he or she might make of such prejudicial actions would give the appearance of oversensitivity and possibly incite further reaction from the initiator. For example, a woman may be placed in an awkward situation when she is congratulated for offering a solution to a technical engineering problem as if such an idea would not be normally expected of a woman. The person targeted by prejudicial actions is not the only person affected. Prejudice affects the behaviour of the person holding the prejudice as well. That person may harbor anxieties or anger, or alter his normal activity because of the prejudice he feels for someone else. Such feelings of prejudice can lead to alcohol and substance abuse just as for people who are the targets of prejudice.

Crime: Loss of self-esteem and hope for future betterment contributes to criminal behavior. Though crime occurs in all classes of society, such as white-collar crime in the upper classes, social class position influences the type of crime that someone will commit. Through violent and property crimes committed by lower classes, not only is there a loss of productivity to the community, but other costs associated with crime include the expenses of police in crime-fighting activity. The percentage of policing funds spent in the world and the percentage of costs of losses from criminal activity triggered by various form of prejudice would be difficult to calculate from crime statistics kept, but they would likely be considerable. Not only does prejudice contribute to criminal behaviour, prejudice also influences how crime is fought.

Domestic Violence: A major consequence of prejudice is violence. The scale of violence can vary greatly, ranging from occurrences of domestic violence to mass murder (genocide). Domestic violence is when a family member, partner, or ex-partner physically or psychologically harms or harasses another family member. Aside from physical contact and child abuse, domestic violence can include intimidation and threats of violence. This intimidation can take the form of stalking (harassing someone by relentlessly pursuing her). Domestic violence is often driven by frustrations of lack of economic opportunity due to prejudice and discrimination, and the resulting feelings of powerlessness.

Social Protests: Prejudice and discrimination leads to organized social protests—and sometimes, confrontations—by the targeted groups. Labor strikes, store boycotts (protests by refusing to do business with someone), sit-ins (when protestors refuse to leave a business or public building until their demands are met), and other tactics of social disorder disrupted business productivity. A major consequence of mass opposition to social or governmental prejudices is the loss of legitimacy of society and its institutions to those victimized by prejudice and discrimination. Laws and social customs that perpetuate prejudice undercut the very validity of the nation's social institutions. Broad conflicts over prejudices can lead to social instability. During these times of peak protest activity, society lives with a tension in which any minor incident could trigger a major explosion of violence.

Feelings:

For this area of influence, there are actually two ways in which your feelings can influence your communication with another person. The first simply refers to the way that you feel on a given day; if you feel well, you'll communicate in one way and if you feel ill you'll communicate in another. Since your well-being fluctuates, it makes sense that the way you communicate will change somewhat with how well you are feeling. If you find yourself experiencing difficulty in communicating due to an illness or other physical stressor, recognizing and acknowledging it, when appropriate, can be very helpful when others might interpret the change in your communication as having something to do with them.

The second aspect related to feelings refers to how you feel about a specific person. When you genuinely like someone, the way you communicate is going to show it. Unfortunately, the same can be said for when you don't like someone.

Environment:

The last area of influence on your communication is your environment. All of us communicate differently in different environments. This is simple enough to observe in everyday life. Do you speak to your colleagues the same way that you do to your friends? Do you talk to strangers with more or less formality than people you know well? Do you talk to your subordinates the same way when your own boss is there as you do when she is not there? As you go through your workday, notice how where you are, what is going on and who else is present may be impacting the way that you communicate.

Recognizing how the environment might be affecting others you communicate with is a skill that can come in handy for you, particularly when you perceive that the environment is having a negative impact on your ability to communicate effectively with someone. This skill will help you to perceive why someone might be communicating in the way that they are. It will also give you a factor that you can alter in order to make the person more comfortable or to establish a level of formality that you feel is important in a particular situation.

EXERCISE

1. Write a short note on perspectives of communication.
2. What is visual perception?
3. How does visual perception affect your communication style?
4. What are the other factors affecting perspectives?
5. What is the effect of the environment on the perspective of any person?
6. How does language affect your perspective to communicate?
7. Explain 'past experiences play an important role in designing your perspective towards life and communication'.
8. Describe 'prejudice has some psychological effect on your perspective to communicate'.

✱✱✱

Chapter ... 4

ELEMENTS OF COMMUNICATION

♦ LEARNING OBJECTIVES ♦

Objectives of communication are:

- *To make the students learn about importance of communication,*
- *To make them able to understand different types of communication,*
- *To know the different ways to develop their personality with the help of their non verbal communication.*

4.1 INTRODUCTION

Communication is an exchange of facts, ideas, opinions, and emotions by two or more persons. Communication transmits information not only about tangible facts and determinable ideas and opinions but also about emotions when a communicator passes on or transmits sound information, he may also intentionally or unconsciously be communicating his attitude or the frame of his mind. When we are communicating or interacting with anyone then it may be face- to-face or face-off, formal or informal, oral or written or digital or even with the help of visuals.

As studied earlier there are few essential elements of communication like sender, receiver, message and medium, and on the basis of mainly nature of message and medium of communication may be categorized into different categories like:

- **Face-to-face Communication:** Communication where sender and receiver are physically present in front of each other, for example – interviews, group discussions, speech, debates etc.
- **Face-off Communication:** Communication where sender and receiver are not in front of each other. They may be communicating through telephone, mobile, teleconferencing etc.
- **Formal Communication:** Communication in which content, language and situation all are formal, for example – official communication, organizational communication, classroom teaching, seminars, conferences, meetings, group discussions etc.

- **Informal Communication:** Communication in which no formality is observed and language used is also informal, for example – communication between and among friends, colleagues, family members etc.

- **Oral Communication:** Communication or interaction done through oral mode, for example – speech, personal interviews, group discussions, general chit chat etc.

- **Written Communication:** Communication done through written mode, for example – answering questions, writing a book, letter, applications, e-mails, notices, social messaging etc.

- **Visual Communication:** It includes facial expressions, gestures, printed pictures, film strips, postures etc. In organizations, visual signals serve as guidelines for employees to make communication sure and instantaneous.

- **Digital Communication:** When computer or digital technology is used for transmitting messages within and outside the organization, it is digital communication.

- **Symbolic Communication:** It involves verbal and non-verbal symbolism to convey meaning. Art and music are forms of symbolic communication used by nurses to facilitate understanding and healing for patients.

- **Meta-communication:** It is communication about communication, so that 'deeper message within a message' can be uncovered and understood. When a patient tells the nurse that he is cool to undergo surgery with his body rigid and sharp voice, a nurse can interpret that he is anxious as evidenced by body language.

Three Modes of Communication:

On the basis of way of delivery of the message communication may be denoted through three modes:

- **Interpersonal Mode:** Students engage in conversation, provide and obtain information, express feeling and emotions, and exchange opinions.

- **Interpretive Mode:** Students understand and interpret written and spoken language on a variety of topics.

- **Presentation Mode:** Students present information, concepts and ideas to an audience of listeners or readers on a variety of topics.

Transfer of information is possible in two ways either by using language or with the help of body movement. It can be verbal and non-verbal communication.

Verbal Communication: It encompasses both how you deliver messages and how you receive them. Communication is a soft skill, and it's one that is important to everyone whether student or teacher, employee or employer, or any sender and receiver. One who can convey information clearly and effectively are highly valued and are also highly benefited in every field of life. What constitutes effective verbal communication depends on the relationships between communication partners and the work context. Verbal communication in a work setting takes place between many different individuals and groups such as co-workers, bosses and subordinates, employees, customers, clients, teachers and students, and speakers and their audiences. Verbal communication occurs in many different contexts including training sessions, presentations, group meetings, performance appraisals, one-on-one discussions, interviews, disciplinary sessions, sales pitches and consulting engagements.

Non-verbal Communication: When you're interviewing for a job, your body language is almost as important as the answers you give to the questions. Employers will evaluate what you do as well as what you say, and you can use your non-verbal communication skills to make the best impression. Most candidates carefully prepare what they will say during interviews and networking meetings. Less attention is typically paid to how messages are communicated. Your interviewing and networking success will be largely determined by how the people you meet respond to what you are saying. Your non-verbal communications can either support the tone of your conversation or leave the interviewer wondering whether you're all talk and no substance. Displaying non-verbal behaviours that are a match for your messages can help you to convince employers that you are genuinely interested in the job and suited for the work. In general, what's most important is to be positive and engaging. If you feel confident about your ability to do the job and know you'll be an asset to the employer, you can show that by your actions as well as your words. In addition to making a hiring decision, employers will also be evaluating your non-verbal skills to determine whether you will be able to relate effectively to clients, co-workers and business associates. In many occupations, the ability to establish credibility and trust is a significant success factor. Positive non-verbal behaviour will enable you to demonstrate your sincerity and engaging personality.

4.2 FACE-TO-FACE COMMUNICATION

Face-to-face interaction is a concept in communication studies describing social interaction carried out without any mediating technology. Face-to-face interaction is defined as the mutual influence of individuals' direct physical presence with his/her body language. Face-to-face interaction is one of the basic elements of the social system, forming a significant part of individual socialization and experience gaining throughout one's lifetime. Similarly it is also central to the development of various groups and organizations composed of those individuals.

Study of face-to-face interaction is defined as the process of recording and analyzing the reactive pattern of individuals when they are involved in a face-to-face interaction. It is concerned with issues such as its organization, rules, and strategy. The concept of face-to-face interaction has been of interest to scholars since at least the early 20th century. One of the earliest social science scholars to analyze this type of interaction was sociologist **Georg Simmel**, who in his 1908 book observed that sensory organs play an important role in interaction, discussing examples of human behaviour such as an eye contact.

Face-to-face communication has been however described as less preferable to mediated communication in some situations, particularly where time and geographical distance are an issue. For example, in maintaining a long-distance friendship, face-to-face communication was only the fourth most common way of maintaining ties, after telephone, email, and instant messaging.

Despite the advent of many new information and communication technologies, face-to-face interaction is still widespread and popular and has a better performance in many different areas where face-to-face communication is described as the most efficient and informational one. This is explained because face-to-face communication engages more human senses than mediated communication. Face-to-face interaction is also a useful way for people when they want to win over others based on verbal communication, or when they try to settle disagreements. Besides, it does help a lot for teachers as one effective teaching method. It is also easier to keep a stronger and more active political connection with others by face-to-face interaction.

Face-to-face communication offers more scope to motivate team members than electronic communication. It also allows you to get a clear picture of how well your message has been understood and whether the team member has any reservations about what they are being asked to do. Face-to-face communication is particularly suitable for discussion as there is immediate feedback from the listener. It is particularly effective when the work under discussion requires coordination and collaboration. One of the biggest advantages of face-to-face communication is that it can create a bond of trust between people in a way that electronic communication simply cannot.

Face-to-face communication may be defined as communication when the communicator transmits his message in person to the receiver in person verbally and even non-verbally. Thus face-to-face communication is both verbal and non-verbal. All face communication is oral, but all oral communication need not to be face-to-face, for example, the telephonic talk is oral but not face-to-face. The types of face-to-face communication are as follows: Interviews, Meetings, Conferences, Seminars, Workshops, Class-room lectures, Stage-acting, Public lectures, etc.

Principles/Dynamics of Effective Face-To-Face Communication:
- In face-to-face communication at least two individuals (receiver and sender) should be physically and mentally present at the place of communication.
- In face-to-face communication there should be proper encoding with most appropriate and pleasing words by sender.
- In face-to-face communication there should be proper decoding by the receiver after receiving the message.
- In face-to-face communication there should be some (partial/full) response or feedback. Since it is direct, great care should be taken in the selection of the words which should be appropriate and polite.

The Advantages of Face-to-face Communication

In this modern age of technologically-driven business, it can be easy to push aside actual, physical human interaction for communication via electronic device. We email, we IM, we use social media, we text, we talk on the phone, but we often forget that all of these are missing one common component – real, face-to-face, human interaction. Therefore, the question must be asked... does it matter? Does face-to-face time with your team really make a difference to them, or are they more than willing to receive their instructions via email and through phone calls?

This is a great question, and is one that holds a lot of relevancy today. We do live in an age of electronic communication, and it does help us in a lot of ways... but has it gone too far? Are many employees feeling disconnected due to a lack human interaction, and is it having detrimental effects on their productivity? To be honest, the answer is different for everyone. There might be people out there who don't mind not speaking face-to-face as often, though the largest percentage of people would benefit from more actual, tangible human interaction... especially where their management is concerned. Now it is discussed 'what are the advantages of face-to-face communication over communication via electronic devices?'

Face-to-face Communication Creates More Motivation: There is no denying the fact that speaking to someone in person can make it much easier to motivate them. Of course, you could write a long-winded message to your employees telling them how much they do for the company, but is this going to be more effective than walking up to them, smiling at them, and thanking them in person for their hard work? While you can definitely contribute to motivating your team through electronic communication, there is no doubt that face-to-face interaction has a special relevance in this area. Face-to-face communication also helps to build collaborative environments that inspire and energize employees to participate in meetings, brainstorming sessions and more. These environments foster engagement and innovation, which is important for employee satisfaction as well as company culture and growth.

Face-to-face Communication Makes it Easier to Sense What a Person is Really Thinking: While it might be possible to 'read' a person based on the language in their emails, there is no greater way to gauge what an individual is thinking than to speak to them in person. Did you know that spoken words account for less than 10% of the communication between humans? The rest consists of body language, voice inflection, facial cues etc. Therefore, it stands to reason that, in order to really communicate with someone on a level that will allow you to 'read' the subtleties in their communication that are not made up of actual words, making sure that there is at least a healthy amount of face-to-face interaction would definitely be a positive thing. Non-verbal cues are just as crucial when communicating as the words we say. Everything from body language and facial expressions to attentiveness and engagement can indicate different thoughts and feelings – each of which can only truly be observed through face-to-face communication.

Face-to-face Communication Creates a Bond: Whether you want to call it friendship, a partnership, camaraderie, or simply a good working relationship, developing a real bond with someone is far more difficult if you do not ever get to speak to them face-to-face. When it comes to your team, you are likely going to need to develop at least a decent amount of trust for each other... so why forgo face-to-face interaction when it could serve to better strengthen the bonds of trust between two people who are going to be relying on each other and working together? Of course, you don't need to be friends with everyone that you work for, but friendship can happen in the workplace, and avoiding face-to-face interaction may definitely impede this natural process from running its course. A sense of community comes with the ability to interact and socialize, and this sets the foundation for trust, and ultimately better working relationships.

Addressing Sensitive Issues: When addressing sensitive issues, put down the phone, move away from the keyboard, and make the effort to engage in-person – it will be crucial to a successful outcome. Whether you are providing specific feedback to a staff member or addressing an issue with a colleague, much can be misinterpreted or lost when communicating via technology. Focus on your desired outcome and prepare by considering the mindset and possible reactions of the one you will be communicating with. This can help to turn a challenging conversation into a trust-building interaction.

Clear and Concise Communication: How many times has an email been misunderstood, misread or perceived by another party to be rude when that wasn't the intention? Face-to-face conversations minimize the risk of miscommunication, promoting more effective business practices. Sometimes encouraging face-to-face interactions can be as simple as persuading others to walk down the corridor rather than sending an email. The importance of real conversations, in real time and real rooms, should never be underestimated.

Today's technology makes communication faster and easier than ever before. But it shouldn't be the only way we communicate. And for all our innovation, nothing can quite replace the impact of face-to-face communication.

Types of Communication:

Communication is an exchange of facts, ideas, opinions, and emotions by two or more persons. Communication transmits information not only about tangible facts and determinable ideas and opinions but also about emotions. When a communicator passes on or transmits sound information, he may also intentionally or unconsciously be communicating his attitude or the frame of his mind. Transfer of information is possible in two ways either by using language or with the help of body movement. Thus, communication can be divided into two classes – verbal and non-verbal.

Verbal Communication is when we communicate our massage verbally. It requires the use of words, vocabulary and symbols. We transfer information which may be factual or specific. It may also convey emotions, attitudes, beliefs, desires etc. A symbol is essentially a sign to which some meaning is assigned by convention rather than by any external similarity between the sign and its denotation. Thus, for example, a word like lion is a symbol: the word does not resemble a lion.

Non-verbal Communication: When we use language of signs, symbols and gestures rather than that of words for communicating or interacting with others it is known as non-verbal communication. The main elements of the non-verbal communication are personal appearance, postures, gestures with different parts of the body, facial expressions, eye contact, the distance between the speaker and the listener, the tone of the speaker, the volume of the speaker, the pauses taken between words and sentences, the emotional content of the communication. All non-verbal cues help the communicator to talk without words. These cues are used to express love, respect, likes, dislikes, dependence, feelings etc. Non-verbal cues give us the following information:

- They interpret human behaviour.
- They transmit our messages.
- They also give clues about intentions, emotions, views, social status and personalities of the people.
- This communication is less deliberate and conscious; rather it is subtle and instinctive as compared to verbal communication.

To make communication effective statistics show that words play only a 7% role, tone of the voice 38% and non-verbal cues play a role of the remaining 55%, show how material is more important that what is said.

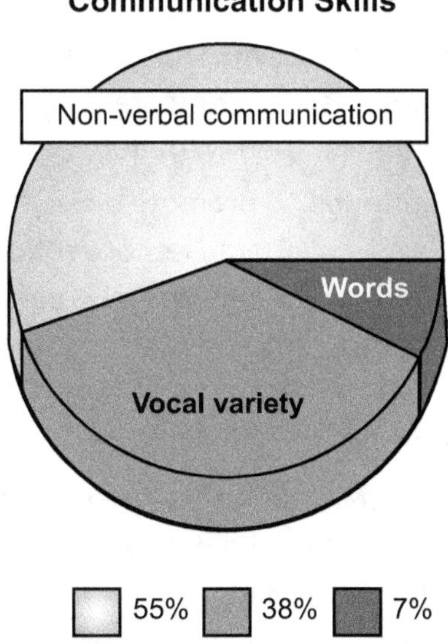

Fig. 4.1: Communication Skills

Verbal communication:

When two people interact by using language, it is known as verbal communication. If we are using oral mode of language for transferring information it is known as oral communication. If we use written mode of language for transferring information, it is known as written communication.

Oral Communication:

It implies the conveying of message through spoken words. It is face-to-face communication between the individuals and also includes communication through telephone, intercom, public speech etc. The important feature of oral communication is that the real meaning is conveyed by the manner or tone of the voice or facial expression of the communicator and the communicatee. There are many methods of oral communication: dyadic communication, telephonic conversation, interview, dictation, meeting, interviewing, lectures, announcements, radio talks, TV and cinema shows, seminars and conferences, group discussions, use of audio visual aids, and negotiations.

Categories of Oral Communication

1. **Discussion:** Its motive is to discuss actions, suggest ideas and come to decisions. Let others speak, listen to others with openness and always be ready to accept their viewpoints, exchange facts and opinions. The purpose is not to win an argument but to come to some constructive conclusion. Discussion must lead towards the right answer.

2. **Debate:** Constructive communication is productive dialogues and skillful discussions where new insights could emerge through healthy give and take. In debate you are visualizing both pros and cones, negative and positive of a situation. Do not try to knock each other out; your opponent may be right in his perspective. Debate should not create a close-minded attitude. Do not listen to find flaws and counter arguments. As compared to discussion, debate tends to be competitive. Always use the competitive nature of debate to your advantage.

3. **Dialogue:** Dialogue is designed to promote a free flowing interchange of ideas and create an open, equal and collaborative conventional climate. The purpose is to share perspective and understanding. We take each other's ideas to develop new ideas and concepts. You can explore issues creatively. Dialogue creates an open-minded attitude.

Merits of Oral Communication

- **It is economical:** Oral communication is economical as compared to written communication, especially if it is within the organization.
- Oral communication is less time consuming.
- **Immediate Feedback:** The biggest advantage of oral communication is that it provides immediate feedback to both the senders and the receivers.

- **It gives the chance for clarification:** Oral communication being face-to-face communication gives the opportunity for clarifications.
- **It has personal touch:** Oral communication is very much in use for informal purposes like to promote friendly relationships between the parties communicating with each other that lead to greater understanding.
- **Communication with larger public:** Oral communication is extremely useful while communicating with groups or large mass or meetings.
- **It is flexible:** Oral communication is flexible in nature. Oral communication provides an opportunity to the speaker to correct himself and make himself clear by changing his voice, pitch, tone etc.

Demerits of Oral Communication

- It is less reliable.
- Not possible to approach distant people in the absence of a mechanical device.
- It is not suitable for lengthy messages.
- Messages cannot be retained for longer duration, hence cannot provide any record for future references.
- It is not having any legal validity.
- There may be comparatively greater chances of misunderstanding.
- It is not easy to fix responsibility in case of misunderstanding or dispute.
- It is influenced by self-interest and attitude of the people.

Written Communication:

Written communication implies transmission of messages in black and white. Everything that is transmitted in the written form falls in the area of written communication. It includes circulars, reports, magazines, manuals, newspapers letters, applications, tenders, memos, notices, telegrams, e-mails, pictures, diagrams, graphs, agreements, rule and procedure books, orders, instructions, questionnaires etc.

Merits of Written Communication

- **Permanent Record:** Written communication has the advantage of being a permanent record of the organization for future reference.
- **Accurate and Precise:** Written communication is the result of serious thinking and planning and also editing, which results in less number of errors.
- **Legal Document:** Written communication is a legal document because of which the merits of the meetings, conferences, discussions etc are jotted down in black and white.
- **Wider Access:** Written communication enjoys wider access because of its frequency. It is the only means used for distant places even beyond telephonic ranges.
- **To Assign Responsibilities:** Written communication is preserved for future references because it becomes easy to assign responsibilities.
- **Composing in Advance:** Written communication can be composed in advance long before it has to be delivered.

- **Referred to Again and Again:** The written messages can be read again and again; therefore the message is likely to be understood better.
- **Mechanical Efficiency:** Messages can be written and conveniently transcribed, transmitted, filed and retrieved.
- **Lengthy Message:** Written communication is very suitable for transmitting lengthy messages. Words can be supplemented with charts, diagrams etc.

Demerits of Written Communication

- It's very time consuming.
- It is very expensive in terms of time, money, energy etc.
- In written communication quick clarification is not possible.
- It becomes difficult to maintain secrecy about a written communication.
- It may be interpreted in a different manner by different people.

4.3 NON-VERBAL COMMUNICATION

Non-verbal language gives us the cues for interpreting human behaviour, for transmitting messages and clues about intentions, emotions, views, personality and social status of the people. In this communication we are concerned with things like body language, postures, gestures, space, tone, voice system. While on a job interview, you might think that if you have the best answers to the interview questions, you'll get the job. In fact, that isn't necessarily the case. A big part of the success of your answers is actually non-verbal communication. This includes your body language and what is known as "paralanguage" – the elements of your speech besides the words, such as your intonation, speaking speed, pauses and sighs, and facial expressions. Non-verbal communication also includes your attire and grooming. Non-verbal communication is as important, or even more important than, verbal communication. The interviewer will be observing your non-verbal communication throughout the entire interview. If your non-verbal communication skills aren't up to par, it won't matter how well you answer the questions.

Non-verbal communication matters as soon as you walk in the office door. If you come to an interview reeking of chewing gum, you will already have one strike against you. Too much perfume or not enough deodorant won't help either. Not being dressed appropriately or having scuffed shoes will give you a second strike. Talking on your cell phone or listening to music while waiting to be called for the interview may be your final strike.

What's important when interviewing is to appear professional, attentive, and confident throughout the interview process. Before you leave for the interview, make sure you are dressed professionally, are neatly groomed, your shoes are polished, and you haven't overdone the perfume or aftershave (none is better than too much).

There are things that you should bring with you to the interview and things that you need to leave at home. What to Bring to an Interview: Portfolio or pad holder with a copy of your resume and a list of references on quality paper, Work samples (if relevant), Notepad and pen; and What Not to Bring to an Interview are: Cell phone, iPod, Gum, Candy, Soda or coffee, Scuffed shoes, messy and/or not-so-clean clothes. The way you sit in the lobby, the way you greet the receptionist and the interviewer, and the way you wait, will all have an impact on whether you are going to be considered for the job. Be friendly and pleasant, but not overbearing. If you need to wait, sit quietly (no phone calls) and patiently.

Shake hands with the interviewer. Your handshake should be firm – not sticky or wimpy. To avoid sweaty palms, visit the rest room, wash your hands, and then run them under cool water prior to the interview. Keep your palms open rather than clenched in a fist and keep a tissue in your pocket to (discreetly) wipe them.

Important non-verbal communications during interview are:

- Make eye contact with the interviewer for a few seconds at a time.
- Smile and nod (at appropriate times) when the interviewer is talking, but don't overdo it. Don't laugh unless the interviewer does first.
- Be polite and keep an even tone to your speech. Don't be too loud or too quiet.
- Don't slouch.
- Do relax and lean forward a little towards the interviewer so you appear interested and engaged.
- Don't lean back. You will look too casual and relaxed.
- Keep your feet on the floor and your back against the lower back of the chair.
- Pay close attention to the interviewer. Take notes if you are worried you will not remember something.
- Don't interrupt.
- Stay calm. Even if you had a bad experience at a previous position or were fired, keep your emotions to yourself and do not show anger or frown.
- Before leaving the interview, be sure to give the interviewer another firm handshake and smile. On your way out, say goodbye to the receptionist or anyone else you spoke to during the interview.
- Of course, your verbal communication is important too. Remember your manners and thank the interviewer for taking the time to meet with you. Don't use slang. Speak clearly and definitely.

We could classify non-verbal communication into four different broad categories: Kinesis or Body language, Proxemics or Personal Space language, Chronemics or time, Paralingual.

Kinesics: Body movement or body language.

Proxemics: Space language.

Chronemics: Time Language.

Paralingual: Actions and words as hints for communication (pitch/voice/manner etc.).

4.4 BODY LANGUAGE OR KINESICS

Kinesis means body language: The communication without words and through various movements of body parts. All the body movements are guided by our thought process, emotions etc. By nodding, blinking and various other ways we send out our signals and messages that often speak louder than words. A body movement consciously or instinctively carries messages, attitudes, moods, feeling and so on. The term body language includes: facial expression, gestures, body movements or postures, eye contact, haptics etc.

(i)   Facial Expressions: Face is the primary site for expressing emotions; it reveals both the type and intensity of the feelings. There is a statement given by Paul Elliman, "We talk with our vocal cords but we communicate with the facial expressions, our tone of voice, our whole body etc. Therefore understanding body language has immense practical use. Facial expressions convey fear, sadness, disgust, liking disliking, rejection, love, frustration, happiness, anger, surprise boredom etc. Thus, if you smile frequently you will be perceived as more likable, friendly, warm and approachable. Smiling is often contagious and a person will react favorably.

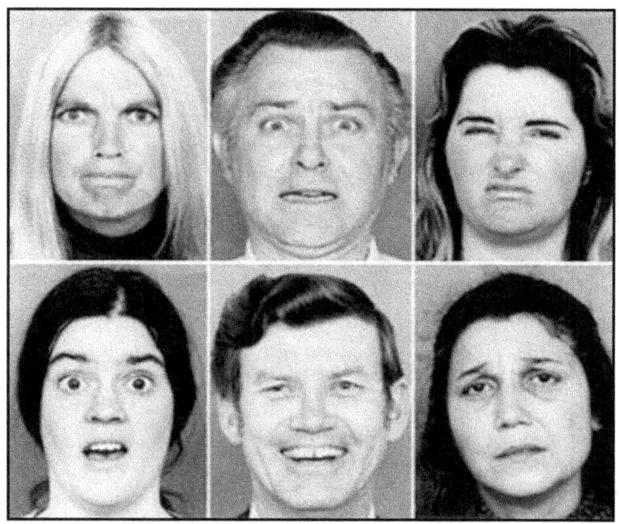

Fig. 4.2: Different Facial Expressions

Four important parts of the human face are: Upper face – forehead and eyebrows; Middle face – the sides of face, cheeks; and Lower face – mouth and chin. These parts of the human face are capable of having a wide range of expressions and emotions.

W. Evary has listed the following possible components of facial expressions:

1.   **Forehead** – upward and downward frown, eyebrows-raising or knitting, furrowing,

2.   **Eyelids –** opening, closing, narrowing,

3.   **Eye pupils** – dilating,

4.   **Eyes –** upwards, downwards, gazing, holding or avoiding eye contact

5. **Nose** – wrinkling, flaring nostrils

6. **Facial muscles** – drawn up or grown

7. **Mouth** – wide open, drawn in and half open

8. **Tongue** – licking lips, moving around inside cheeks, sucking teeth

9. **Jaw, Chin** – thrust forward, handing down

10. **Head** – thrown back, inclines to one side hanging down chin, drawn in, inclined upward etc.

(ii) Gesture: A gesture is a non-vocal bodily movement intended to express meaning. They may be articulated with the hands, arms or body, and also include movements of the head, face and eyes, such as winking, nodding, or rolling one's eyes. The boundary between language and gesture, or verbal and non-verbal communication can be hard to identify. If you fail to gesture while speaking, you may be perceived as boring, stiff and unanimated. Gestures mean motion of head, hand or body itself, to express an idea or emotion or feeling. Examples – sitting positions, eye signals, hand shake, head nod, collar pull, thumbs up, thumb and finger rub, shoulder shrug, blink of the eye.

(iii) Posture or Body Movement: Body movement, speeches to others, postures give us an idea about the attitude of the hearer to impart involvement in communication. Posture indicates superiority, confidence, anxiety, and rejection. Facial expression and body movement states that a person tends to lean forward when he is involved or interested and to lean back when not interested. The way of talking often indicates to others whether feeling good, happy, cheerful, sad, gloomy, tired, rejected etc. Your posture – including the pose, stance and bearing of the way you sit, slouch, stand, lean, bend, hold and move your body in space affects the way people perceive you. Studies investigating the impact of posture on interpersonal relationships suggest that mirror-image congruent postures, where one person's left side is parallel to the other's right side, leads to favorable perception of communicators and positive speech; a person who displays a forward lean or a decrease in a backwards lean also signify positive sentiment during communication.

Difference between Gesture and Posture

A gesture is a form of non-verbal communication in which visible bodily actions communicate particular messages, whereas posture is a stance and/or alignment as compared to a balanced position for the human body. Body language is the non-verbal, usually unconscious, communication through the use of postures, gestures, facial expressions, and the like. A gesture is a form of non-verbal communication in which visible bodily actions communicate particular messages, either in place of speech or together and in parallel with spoken words. Gestures include movement of the hands, face, or other parts of the body. Gestures differ from physical non-verbal communication that does not communicate specific messages, such as purely expressive displays, proxemics, or displays of joint attention. Gestures allow individuals to communicate a variety of feelings and thoughts, from contempt and hostility to approval and affection, often together with body language in addition to words when they speak.

(iv) Eye Contact or Oculosis: The eyes speak with an eloquence and truthfulness. It is the window out of which the wings of thought often fly unwillingly. The eye contact is of paramount importance in all facial expressions. When we look at somebody's face we focus primarily on his eyes and try to understand what it means. The language of the eye contact serves as a signal or readiness to interact and its absence tends to reduce the chances of such interaction. Usually the person who seeks eye contact is regarded as honest and self-confident, or negative or poor eye contact rejects lack of confidence. Eye contact can indicate interest, attention, and involvement. Furthermore, eye contact with audiences increases the speaker's credibility. Gaze comprises the actions of looking while talking, looking while listening, amount of gaze, and frequency of glances, patterns of fixation, pupil dilation, and blink rate.

(v) Haptics or Touch: It is the easiest or one of the easiest forms of human communication. Touches that can be defined as communication include handshake, holding hands, kissing (cheek, lips, and hand), back slapping, give five, a pat on the shoulder, and brushing an arm. The meaning conveyed from touch is highly dependent upon the context of the situation, the relationship between communicators, and the manner of touch. Stroking, hitting, patting and shaking hands etc. are the important modes and play a role in human behaviour. A gentle touch of a friendly hand on the shoulders can communicate encouragement; a limp, a handshake, indicates lack of interest.

Proxemics or Personal Space Language:

It refers to the non-verbal study of space and distance we use to communicate a message. The concept of territorial space refers to the area around the self that a person will not allow another person to enter without consent. Human relationships can be characterized as intimate, personal, social and public. The way people communicate with one another depends upon the proxemics where the people are in relation to one another. How we interact with our physical space can communicate a lot to other people. Are we friendly? Are we mean? Are we possibly insane? One of the basic ideas in communication is immediacy, or the ways that we communicate openness, friendliness, and a desire or willingness to communicate with others. Just think about it, how do you signal to someone that you are interested in communicating?

Common non-verbal signals of immediacy include things like smiling and waving, but this also extends to your use of physical space. Again imagine two people in a room together, one with his back to the other, leaning against a wall with his arms crossed. The other is taking up more physical space, displaying an openness and trustfulness. Which of these people is showing more immediacy? The one taking up more physical space is communicating immediacy. Immediacy is what we use when we want to display openness. But, sometimes we want to communicate something else, like what's ours. Territoriality is the non-verbal communication of ownership. When you feel protective of a specific physical space or item, your body language reflects that.

Again imagine two figures of people using non-verbal cues to denote ownership. The first person is sitting on a couch, but is stretched out all across it, taking up as much space as possible. If that person was interested in sharing this space, he'd be sitting on it differently. Figure two is sitting at a table, and is demonstrating her territoriality by filling up the space on the table with her papers, books, and coffee. Again, the message is clear: 'I'm using this space, don't touch.'

Most of our interaction with the world around us is defined by personal space, the immediate area around a person through which they feel ownership and safety. Our personal space is very important to us. Think of this as your personal bubble. You don't like just anybody coming inside your bubble; this can make you feel insecure, possible unsafe, and generally irritable.

We expect people to respect our personal space, and when they don't, we can react with hostility. This is called expectations violation theory. Basically, the idea is that we have expectations about personal space that are generally cultural, and we will use non-verbal communication to express discomfort or dissatisfaction when those expectations aren't met. For many people, this is one of the major areas of culture shock when travelling, since different cultures have very different ideas about personal space.

In order to prevent this from happening, most of us try to non-verbally communicate the extent of our bubbles to everyone around us. We call the creation of a protective buffer zone around a person the body buffer zone. Basically, this is another way to describe the personal bubble. You create a buffer zone, the limits of your personal space, and when people move into it, you find ways to communicate discomfort. The further into the buffer zone they get, the less subtle those signs are.

Proxemics is another notable area in the non-verbal world of body language and is related to spatial relationships. Introduced by Edward T. Hall in 1966, proxemics is the study of measurable distances between people as they interact with one another. Hall also came up with four distinct zones in which most men operate. According to this buffer zone or proxemics, the distance zones may be:

- **Intimate:** (Up to 2 feet), most sensitive zone, since it is reserved for close friends, and loved   ones. Intimate distance for embracing, touching or whispering; Close phase – less than 6 inches (15 cm) and Far phase – 6 to 18 inches (15 to 46 cm).

- **Personal:** (2 to 4 feet) Personal distance for interactions among good friends or family members; Close phase – 1.5 to 2.5 feet (46 to 76 cm) and Far phase – 2.5 to 4 feet (76 to 122 cm).

- **Social:** (4 to 12 feet) Social distance for interactions among acquaintances; Close phase – 4 to 7 feet (1.2 to 2.1 m) and Far phase – 7 to 12 feet (2.1 to 3.7 m).

- **Public:** (greater than 12 feet) Public distance used for public speaking; Close phase – 12 to 25 feet (3.7 to 7.6 m) and Far phase – 25 feet (7.6 m) or more.

In addition to physical distance, the level of intimacy between conversants can be determined by "socio-petal socio-fugal axis", or the "angle formed by the axis of the conversants' shoulders". Changing the distance between two people can convey a desire for intimacy, declare a lack of interest, or increase/decrease domination. It can also influence the body language that is used. For example, when people talk they like to face each other. If forced to sit side by side, their body language will try to compensate for this lack of eye-to-eye contact by leaning in shoulder-to-shoulder.

It is important to note that as with other types of body language, proximity range varies with culture. Hall suggested that "physical contact between two people ... can be perfectly correct in one culture, and absolutely taboo in another". In Latin America, people who may be complete strangers may engage in very close contact. They often greet one another by kissing on the cheeks. North Americans, on the other hand, prefer to shake hands. While they have made some physical contact with the shaking of the hand, they still maintain a certain amount of physical space between the other persons. In India we try to avoid any kind of close proximity with strangers.

Chronemics:

It involves the meaning given to time dimension when we are communicating to someone. Delay in replying to a personal or business letter or a phone call, coming late for work or meetings are example of chronemics. In non-verbal communication completion of task within a specific time span is recommended; it communicates hard work, sincerity, and loyalty.

Paralanguage:

It involves the 'how' of the sender's voice or the manner in which he speaks. Paralanguage (sometimes called vocalics) is the study of non-verbal cues of the voice. Various acoustic properties of speech such as tone, pitch and accent, can all give off non-verbal cues. Paralanguage may change the meaning of words. Different elements of paralanguage are pitch variation, speaking speed, volume variation, tone variation, pauses between words and sentences, proper words' stress, the clearness of the voice etc.

1.   Pitch variation: It is very important to keep the listener's attention to the speaker's content. It has been observed that people in authority speak in a high-pitched voice while juniors use low- pitched voice. Emotions also affect our pitch; if we are in anger, distress, anxiety our pitch automatically increases.

2.   Speaking speed: We speak at different speeds on different occasions. Easiest part of the message could be spoken at a brief pace, difficult or complicated or technical part of the message should be spoken at a slower pace.

3.   Volume variation: The voice should be loud enough so that it reaches the audience comfortably and loudness can be adjusted according to the situation.

4.   Proper Word Stress: It is of crucial importance in communication, just by changing the stress on different words of the same sentence their meaning could be changed. For example:

- 'Please give me my book.
- Please 'give me my book.
- Please give 'me my book.
- Please give me 'my book.
- Please give me my 'book.

In the first sentence the speaker is requesting to get his book. In sentence 2, the speaker wants his book back. In sentence 3, the speaker wants to get his book back (and it should be given to him only not to anybody else). In sentence 4 the speaker wants to get back his own book (not of anybody else). In sentence 5, the speaker wants to get back his book (not anything else).

Key Points Regarding Body Language:

Body language or non-verbal signals tell us about the person's attitude, outlook, interests, and approach. They speak louder than the verbal communication during the interview or any type of interaction. "The most important thing in communication is hearing what isn't said."   **– Peter F. Drucker**

The non-verbal communication helps to confidently assess each candidate's credentials with regard to the skills necessary to do the job, behavioural characteristics you have identified as necessary for success in the job, and culture and environment of the organization.

These are examples of non-verbal communication you need to pay attention to and "hear."

- **First Impressions:** The first few minutes in any interview setting are so important that almost nothing else matters. Observer takes a look at the candidate and notes all of the non-verbal messages one is communicating. Interviewers form impressions from the candidate's posture, handshake, outfit and accessories, space usage, attentiveness, eye contact, and facial expressions. And, then listen to what candidate has to say in response to the questions.

- **Posture and Space Usage:** Is the candidate sitting comfortably yet upright, but not stiffly, in his chair? Does he walk with a self-assured ease? He's likely confident and comfortable with himself. Slouchy posture speaks loudly about sloppy work and low self-esteem. Posture that enables an individual to take up the appropriate amount of space in the room tells you that the applicant is secure in his abilities. Sloppy posture gives the impression of low energy and carelessness. Pay attention.

- **Handshake:** Notice whether the candidate has a firm, dry, solid handshake. Again, a confident, comfortable person uses the handshake as a positive non-verbal interaction. The handshake should assure you of the candidate's desire for a positive first interaction and impression. A limp handshake signals low confidence and low self-esteem. An excessively strong handshake may tell you the person is overly aggressive or trying to steamroll you.

- **Clothing and Accessories:** No matter how informal the work environment is, a professional job candidate needs to wear a suit/saree to her first meeting. The selected outfit tells how well the candidate will interact with and be perceived by customers. The chosen accessories either telegraph professionalism – or they don't. A briefcase, a leather portfolio, a nice pen, leather purse and shined shoes present a solid, professional appearance.

- Makeup, perfume, and jewelry, worn tastefully, can add to the perception of their professionalism. Dirty fingernails or scuffed shoes tells or indicates that the person is careless, too hurried, or unaware of the impression they have on others. And it is not good.

- **Attentiveness and Eye Contact:** Watch the listening and interactive behaviour of the candidate. He should act as if he is engaged by leaning slightly forward in his chair to close some of the distance between himself and the interviewer. Everybody wants an employee who can maintain comfortable eye contact without staring or forced attentiveness. If the candidate spends the interview with his eyes moving all over the room, rarely looking at you, this can signal a lack of confidence – or worse – he doesn't care. Long, forced eye contact can indicate an overly aggressive person who does not care about your comfort. And, if he doesn't care about the comfort during the interview, that behaviour won't get better when you hire him.

- **Listen also to the candidate's responses to the questions:** Did he hear your question? Did he answer succinctly and share stories, or ramble incessantly off topic? The former tells you he prepared for the interview and has success stories to share. The latter signals unprepared, ill-at-ease, or that he didn't care enough to pay attention.

- **Facial Expressions and Body Language:** "What you do speaks so loud that I cannot hear what you say," said Ralph Waldo Emerson. And, nothing is as communicative as the facial expressions and body language of your candidates. Facial expressions that fail to match the words spoken can indicate serious discomfort or lying – neither desirable behaviours in a candidate. A candidate that never makes eye contact and talks to a spot over your shoulder is uncomfortable and demonstrating a lack of confidence. You want to hire an employee whose facial expressions are consistent with and punctuate her words.

- Body language speaks loudly, too. Is the candidate leaning back in his seat with his legs crossed at the knee? He's too relaxed for an interview setting. Has he taken over your whole desk with his arms and accessories? He's overly aggressive. Does he lean back with his hands crossed behind his head? This is aggressive interview behaviour in the extreme. Don't expect less aggressive behaviour if you hire him.

- If the candidate makes a statement and looks away from you or appears nervous, she's probably not telling the truth. If she stares into your eyes as she tells her story, she may be fabricating.

- If she taps her pen constantly, twists her jewelry at the end of every sentence, strokes her hair every few minutes, she is sending all sorts of messages about her discomfort – with the interview setting or with her skills and abilities in general.

Listening to the non-verbal communication of your candidates can tell you as much about the candidates as their spoken words, their references, and their experience. Non-verbal communication matters.

4.5 TONE OF VOICE

Tone, in linguistics, is a variation in the pitch of the voice while speaking. Tone is the attitude or how somebody sounds whereas intonation is the rise and fall of voice, sound or tone. Tone is shown or heard in how something is being said. It is more like an attitude rather than being a voice pattern. It is somebody's general sound; he may sound happy, upset, excited, angry or ecstatic among other moods. Thus, tone is part of pragmatic communication. This means that emotion has a great deal of influence to one's tone. By using different tones, the words in a sentence can have other meanings aside from the real original meaning of those words.

Tone of voice is the quality of a person's voice. Tone of voice shows manner of speaking, delivery and speech – or we can say it is your characteristic style or manner of expressing yourself orally. A tone of voice also shows what the speaker is feeling; for example; there was a note of uncertainty in his voice; he spoke in a nervous tone of voice; there is a musky roundness to his wordiness; he spoke in undertones etc. One can adjust one's tone by fluctuating the pitch. When your pitch increases in a particular manner it's called rising intonation. When your pitch decreases in a particular manner it's called falling intonation.

A study by Dr. Mehrabian investigated the impact when words and other communication were not consistent. Findings showed that only 7% of the message people received was dependent on the words you use. 38% reflected tone of voice and 55% facial expression or body language. It's important to know how your tone and appearance affect how people perceive your message. Their perception is reality. As we know the tone of voice we use is responsible for about 35-40 percent of the message we are sending. Tone involves the volume you use, the level and type of emotion that you communicate and the emphasis that you place on the words that you choose.

Tone of Voice in Speaking / Speech:

To see how this works, try saying the sentences below with the emphasis each time on the word in bold –

I didn't say he borrowed my book.

I **didn't** say he borrowed my book.

I didn't **say** he borrowed my book.

I didn't say **he** borrowed my book.

I didn't say he **borrowed** my book.

I didn't say he borrowed **my** book.

I didn't say he borrowed my **book**.

The same sentence can have multiple meanings depending on which word is emphasized. The emphasis on a particular word implies additional information than what the words say. Notice that the meaning of the sentence changes each time, even though the words are the same. The emphasis you place on the word draws the listener's attention, indicating that the word is important somehow. In this case, the emphasis indicates that the word is an error. So in the first example, **I** didn't say he borrowed my book, the phrase includes the message that someone else said it. The implied information continues to change in each sentence, despite the words remaining the same each time.

Tone of Voice in Writing / Literature:

Tone of voice is a combination of spoken language and body language. In literature, the tone of voice refers to the author's feelings towards the subject, as expressed through the writing itself. Tone is more than just the words we choose. It's the way in which we communicate our personality. Tone of voice is the way we tell our users how we feel about our message, and it will influence how they'll feel about our message, too. Despite its name, tone of voice isn't just about how you speak. It includes all the words you use in your business content, including in your notices, sales emails, product brochures, call-center scripts, and client presentations, to name just a few examples. Oh, and by the way, tone of voice isn't the same as good writing or strong messaging. It's the next level up from those things. It's about using language to give your brand its own distinct and recognizable voice.

All the content you produce should have the same tone of voice. When your tone is consistent, your audience hears the same person speaking whenever and however they deal with you. That shows them you're a consistent, reliable company to deal with, and that every part of their experience with you will be equally good. The manner in which something is said can affect how it should be interpreted. Shouting, smiling, irony and so on may add a layer of meaning which is neither pure body language nor speech.

Tone of voice isn't what we say but how we say it. It's the language we use, the way we construct sentences, the sound of our words and the personality we communicate. It is to writing what logo, colour and typeface are to branding. Tone of voice is how the character of your business comes through in your words, both written and spoken. It's not about what you say, but rather the way that you say it, and the impression it makes on everyone who reads or hears you. Think about it. Everyone you meet has their own way of expressing themselves that's as unique as their face or fingerprint. Some are pleasant and polite. Others are pushy and in your face. Some say so much with just a few words. Others never seem to get to the point. Companies are no different.

The difference between voice, tone and style: Tone, voice, and style as three separate elements, which work together in harmony:

Voice is a description of the unique, distinctive voice of your brand. This should cover its personality: is it playful, cheeky and fun like innocent, or personal, inspiring, straightforward and active like Macmillan; its rhythm and pace: are you short and sharp like Oxfam, or musical like Penhaligons; its vocabulary: plain and simple like Ovo, or rich and poetic like Dom Perignon?

Tone is how to use your voice in different situations. In life, we adjust our tone according to who we're talking to and what we're talking about, but our voice remains the same. Your brand voice is singular, but you can use it with many different tones. Separating voice and tone means you can be empathetic to your users, and I think empathy is what makes the difference between just meeting user needs and really engaging them.

Style is a house style for what your writing looks like, for example where to use capitals, how to spell certain words, reminders on grammar, vocabulary. This might also include design elements like how to use, logo, fonts and images. "Be consistent. Be authentic. Be unique."

Remember that you can always vary your tone to fit the situation. Keep your personality consistent, but vary the tone to fit the user's emotional state and the topic. (For example, a company's financial report will need to sound different than the same company's careers page targeted at university students.) You might decide on a casual tone for your site-wide content strategy, but vary the amount of humor in your copy across the site.

The Four Dimensions of Tone of Voice: There are four primary tone-of-voice dimensions.

1. **Funny vs. serious:** Is the writer trying to be humorous? Or is the subject approached in a serious way?
2. **Formal vs. casual:** Is the writing formal? Informal? Casual?
3. **Respectful vs. irreverent:** Does the writer approach the subject in a respectful way? Or does she take an irreverent approach? (In practice, most irreverent tones are irreverent about the subject matter, in an effort to set the brand apart from competitors. They are not usually intentionally irreverent or offensive to the reader.)
4. **Enthusiastic vs. matter-of-fact:** Does the writer seem to be enthusiastic about the subject? Is the organization excited about the service or product, or the information it conveys? Or is the writing dry and matter-of-fact?

Let us see one example using all these four tones of voices. At the core of every piece of writing is the message, the information we're trying to communicate to our user. In this case, our message is, "An error has occurred." Our tone will be how we communicate that message.

First, let's try a serious, formal, respectful, and matter-of-fact error message. "We apologize, but we are experiencing a problem."

Let's make this same message a little more casual. "We're sorry, but we're experiencing a problem at our end."

Let's add a little more enthusiasm to the message. "Oops! We're sorry, but we're experiencing a problem at our end."

If we add an attempt at humor and a little irreverence, we'll have taken the same message to a totally different tone of voice. "What did you do!? You broke it! Just kidding! We're experiencing a problem at our end.)

Tone of Voice in Business:

It was Albert Mehrabian who came up with the rule determining that successful communication is made up of three parts: the words you use, your tone of voice and your body language. Take into consideration the fact that your customers are unable to see your body language through their computer or mobile screen and it's fair to say that tone of voice is the major contributor when writing content.

A tone of voice is an expression of a company's values and way of thinking, and it's not to be considered lightly. Just how the tone of your partner's voice when speaking can instigate hurt feelings, or even an argument, the wrong tone of voice in your content can also put off potential customers.

It tells consumers who you are: Toning a voice gives you the opportunity to advertise your best self. If the kinds of customers you want to attract are businessmen and women, your tone might be authoritative and professional, but if you're targeting teenagers, then it should be more light-hearted and quirky. Having that same consistent tone over time is what will help build your personal brand, and make it likeable. Just don't lie; if you're not a fun brand, don't try to be. There are many types of tones of voice; choose one that reflects your genuine values.

It's what makes you different: Communicating passionately, quietly or angrily can completely impact how people interpret you. If voice and tone was not considered, everybody's business would seem like it was run by the same dull people. And your amazing, innovative, unique business wouldn't be distinguishable from any other. Tone of voice can demonstrate your warmth, expertise, sense of humor, or any other attribute that you want to display to consumers and sets you apart from your competition.

It helps to build trust: When customers identify a tone of voice, they're also identifying a personality. They start to form an image of a person or company based on the tone of voice you present. By doing this, customers feel like they're getting to know the brand or company, bringing with it a sense of trust and familiarity. Developing a consistent tone of voice across all of your customers' connections to your brand, including all social media channels, makes you seem genuine and your customers feel at ease. That familiarity is comforting, as they then know what to expect from you.

It can be used to influence and persuade: Once you have gained the trust of your potential customers, you can use this to influence their decisions and persuade them into doing business with you. After all, they are more likely to do business with a company they like and trust.

So, it makes good business sense to find out who you are as a company and reflect that in your tone of voice communication. Once you pinpoint your values and how you'd like to be perceived, you must make sure all your touch points refer back to these values. Some companies go as far as to create brand guidelines. These help to maintain a consistent look and sound for both consumers and employees and help take a business from being just a company to becoming a brand. Take a look at these inspiring branding guides.

4.6 PHYSICAL COMMUNICATION

Communication is the act of conveying information to a recipient who understands the information and provides appropriate feedback. There are three forms of communication which are verbal communication, written communication and non-verbal communication.

Non-verbal communication is also termed as physical communication. It is a form of communication where symbols, signs and gestures are used. Unlike verbal communication which involves the use of sound and the ear for hearing, physical communication involves the use of the eyes for seeing and other parts of the body for gesturing. Everyone possesses some form of physical communication skills. These include our body posture when speaking, eye contact, facial expressions, touch etc. Even little children know that nodding the head means yes and shaking the head means no. Aside these and some very common gestures, there is more to physical communication skills.

Importance of Physical Communication

Physical communication is as important as any other form of communication. Although it is often under-valued, it is equally as essential as being able to speak or hear. It compliments verbal communication and yields marvelous results when combined effectively with it. In certain professions and job positions, your ability to use physical communication is very important.

- In sporting games, the ability to use and understand signs and gestures is a necessary skill. Coaches and players use them.
- In security agencies, this is a very important skill to possess due to the nature of their operations. The police, navy, military etc. make great use of these skills to avoid being detected by their enemies. Detectives and investigators use some of these non-verbal signs to detect whether a person is lying or telling the truth.
- In the mining and construction industries as well as other work places, where extremely loud sounds hinder verbal communication, physical communication is put to maximum use.
- Counselors, motivational speakers, and public relations officers etc. use physical communication skills when addressing audiences. Great orators do not only speak eloquently but they possess physical communication skills that help draw the attention of their audience.

How to Improve On Physical Communication Skills

Sometimes a person's gestures, facial expressions etc. convey a message that is contrary to what they are saying. Everyone wants their physical communication to reflect exactly what they are trying to say.

Below are a few tips that can help you improve upon your physical communication skills:

Improve on stress management: Our bodies react to stress. These signs of tiredness and frustrations etc. are hard to hide. To avoid exhibiting some of these unwanted physical communication signs take a break in-between work or speeches.

Control anxiety: Just as people can say the wrong words at an interview due to anxiety, anxiety can cause people to exhibit unwanted physical communication signals. Make sure you deal with any anxiety problem before you begin communicating. If you realize you feel tensed, you can take a walk, take in a deep breath or have a cool drink to calm your nerves.

Eye-contact: Establish an eye contact with listeners when communicating. It is a way of expressing your confidence. It is also a way of communicating to a speaker that you are paying attention to him.

Ask for meanings: There are certain body languages that you may never understand until you ask about them. If you do not understand the gestures and facial expressions a person uses, ask them what they mean.

Practice: Consistently practicing your own non-verbal signs and reading other people's gestures will help improve your physical communication skills. We say a person can read people when he understands humans and can interpret their use of gestures.

EXERCISE

1. How is face-to-face communication different from face-off communication?
2. How can the medium play an important role in categorizing communication into different categories?
3. What is visual communication?
4. What is the importance of face-to-face communication for technical students?
5. What is effective communication?
6. What is the difference between oral and written communication?
7. What are the merits and demerits of written communication?
8. What is physical communication?
9. What are the key points of body language which are being observed during an interview?
10. How does verbal communication differ from non-verbal communication?
11. What is the importance of eye contact during oral presentation?
12. What is the difference between gesture and posture?
13. Explain tone of voice in detail.
14. "Your face is very important site of expressions". Explain this statement with various examples.
15. Write short notes on the following topics:

    Proxemics, Chronemics, Tone of Voice, Oculosis, Handshake.

Chapter ... 5

COMMUNICATION STYLES

♦ LEARNING OBJECTIVES ♦

Objectives of this chapter are:
- *To make the students learn different styles of communication.*
- *To make them understand the characteristics of different communication styles.*
- *To make them able to behave accordingly and deal with the people of different communication styles.*

5.1 INTRODUCTION

Effective communication is essential to a happy and productive work environment. The people within a workplace of any size need to feel that there are strong lines of communication that exist within the organization. Managers and employees should be allowed to speak to each other and receive information from each other in useful and supportive ways. A communication style is the way we share information with others. Although we may like to think that we say exactly what we mean and are understood and well received, that may not always be the case. How well our messages come across can depend on the style of communication we use.

There are four different forms of communication: verbal, paraverbal, body language, and personal space. Each form of communication can add to the complexity of communicating. If you can control and understand your own communication form you will be a good communicator. To become an excellent, highly effective communicator, you need to understand other people's communication styles.

Verbal: You have complete control over the words you use in a statement. Differences in age, experience, and background can result in different interpretation of the same statement. It is important that you understand your style and the style of other individuals, so you can better adapt your communication.

Paraverbal: It is not just what you say, but the way you say it that can change the meaning of your statement. The voice tone and intensity, as well as the speed that someone speaks and the pauses in between are examples of paraverbals.

Body Language: It is communicated to others by your body movements and facial expressions. For example, the way you stand, walk, shake hands, and maintain eye contact are all forms of body language.

Personal Space: It includes not only the space between you and others, but also your personal appearance, your choice of decorations, and how you arrange your workspace.

There are four different types of communication styles: direct, spirited, considerate, and systematic. Each style utilizes the four forms of communication differently. Find out what style you are and start being a better communicator.

Although there are four style of communication even then you may need to flex your style in certain situations and with certain people. For example, if your boss has a very direct style, learn to approach meetings with her with a similar direct style...get straight to the point. Think about your personal communication style and the styles of those you work closely with. Are styles getting in the way of business success? Given the importance of communication and the impact it has on your success, paying more attention to it is a vital investment of your time and energy.

5.2 DIRECT COMMUNICATION STYLE

The Direct style (high assertiveness and low expressiveness) characterized by a decisive tone and an emphasis on the bottom line. People with direct style are in control of their lives and decisive in their actions, they thrive on competition. Enjoy challenges but enjoy to win even more. They are with fast pace and single-minded with their goals. Possess strong leadership styles and gets things done at a fast pace. Not afraid to take risks to get what they want.

Direct communication is speech that conveys clear messages or that clearly directs actions. Direct communication is often used in the workplace to ensure clarity regarding who has the authority to give orders and what the orders are. Direct communication may be used when there is no room for discussion or compromise. This style usually doesn't allow the listener to respond with an opinion or viewpoint. For example, your supervisor may say to you, 'You need to get to work on time every day. You must not be late again.' That's pretty direct, right? There's little to no room for misunderstanding what your supervisor means.

Consider how this message might differ if the supervisor chose to convey this message more indirectly, in a way that did not communicate an absolutely clear message or order you to do a clearly specified thing. Suppose that your supervisor says to you, 'Please be mindful of your arrival time every day.' You may be aware of the fact that you are sometimes 15 minutes or so late to work, and your supervisor's words may indicate to you that she doesn't like you being late. But, she has gone about conveying her message to you by way of indirect communication in a way that's somewhat vague or that only implies ideas.

You could very well interpret your supervisor's statement that you should 'be mindful of your arrival time every day' as a suggestion to be aware of exactly when you arrive, and perhaps to make up any time that you miss by working later in the day, for example. The less clear, indirect message from the supervisor may be more pleasant to receive, but it does not communicate a concrete or obvious idea or directive.

People who are direct communicators often tell it like it is. Because of this, they can sometimes appear to be argumentative, aggressive, or just plain rude. Keep in mind that I used the word 'appear.' It is certainly the case that direct communicators may be very nice, caring people. Their behavior may be driven by the desire to achieve an objective or by a passion for what they do.

Consider an example in which two coworkers, Karan and Nischal are trying to finish up a project that they will have to present to their manager soon. Karan may say to Nischal, 'Get the proposal conclusion done by tonight so that we can present it tomorrow.' This statement would be an example of direct communication because it conveys an unambiguous message and clearly directs an action. It's possible that Nischal may not like Karan's blunt order. At the same time, he may appreciate that he understands exactly what Karan's goal is and what part of the job she wants him to complete.

5.3 SPIRITED COMMUNICATION STYLE

The Spirited style (high assertiveness and high expressiveness) , which has an animated style and can be very persuasive. They are enthusiastic and friendly, rather be around other of people then alone. They are able to motivate and generate excitement in others because of their optimistic, focus and lively nature. They thrive in the spot-light of a group of people. They work at a fast pace and are suited for high-profile public position. Fast to build relationships and use their alliances to accomplish work. They are spontaneous and quick to take decisive action.

5.4 SYSTEMATIC COMMUNICATION STYLE

The Systematic style (low assertiveness and low expressiveness) characterized by a precise speaking style with an emphasis on facts. They prefer to make decisions based on facts, not emotions and are very accurate and objective and always rely on data and are excellent problem solvers. Orderly and prefer to work in an organized environment with clear guidelines. Thrive in task-oriented positions that require independent work.

5.5 CONSIDERATE COMMUNICATION STYLE

The Considerate style (low assertiveness and high expressiveness) is a style that features people who listen well and use supportive language. Person with this style value warm personal relationships, good counseling skills and are a good listener. They are cooperative and enjoy being part of a team. They are always aware of others' feelings, and reliable. They are also suitable for any profession that requires you to care for others.

People who are the most comfortable with considerate communication style generally fall under the category of being nice. Strengths of Considerate communicators are that they are; good listeners, build strong relationships on trust, appreciative of others, reliable, patient, and easy to get along with, strong team players. Even then trouble spots of considerate communicators are; have trouble prioritizing, have trouble making decisions, not delegate well, tell you what you want to hear rather than the reality, picks up slack for everyone, places too much emphasis on feelings. Considerate people are great team players. They are also known as the glue that holds the team together. However, they are not able to give accurate feedback which could keep a person under the false impression that everything they are doing is great. Also, they pick up your slack which might deprive you of an opportunity to show what you can do. Considerate people also have a hard time adapting to change. These are all qualities that hinder the considerate people as well as all of them around them. Tips to communicate with people whose dominant style is considerate are ; have one on one conversation with them, be cooperative, listen to them just like they listen to you, build a trust based relationship with them, tell them about changes early on so that they can take their time to adapt to them.

People have vastly diverse communication styles, and not all are compatible. That is, how one says something may not be the best way to communicate to a person or group. Or you may hear what someone says, but not necessarily what they mean. Basically, everyone may interpret the same message in very different ways, possibly resulting in conflict or failure of communication.

DIRECT	SPIRITED	CONSIDERATE	SYSTEMATIC
• Gets to the bottom line. • Speaks forcefully. • Maintains eye contact. • Presents position strongly.	• Persuasive • Is a good story-teller. • Focuses on the big picture. • Uses motivational speech.	• Listens well • Is a good counselor. • Uses supportive language. • Builds trust.	• Presents precisely. • Focus on facts. • Efficient on speech. • Well organized workplace.

5.6 THE MATRIX OF COMMUNICATION STYLES

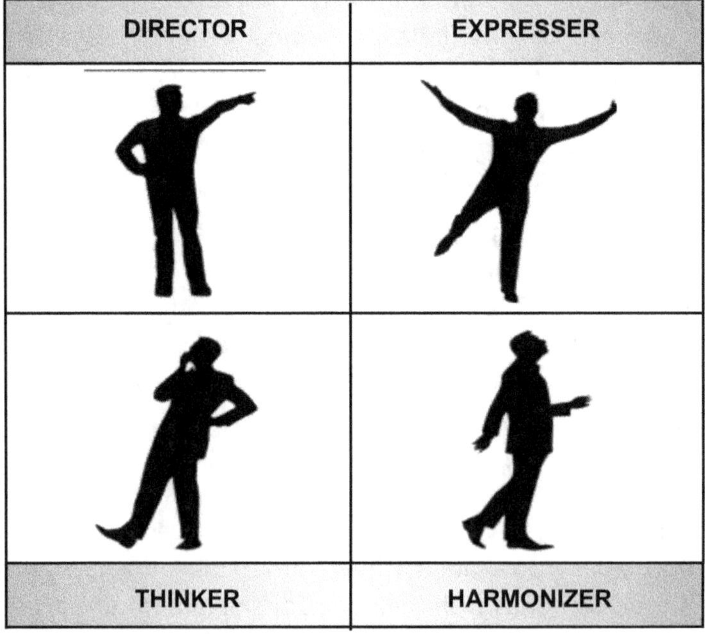

Fig. 5.1

Understanding ones style of communicating would be relatively easy if one limits oneself to one of the four basic styles. However, depending on the situation, one may alternate between one, two, or even three styles. It's like walking. One may naturally walk at a certain pace. But then he shifts gears to match the pace of someone next to him.

It's the same with communicating. People prefer to use one style. Our "primary style" is the one we're most comfortable with. But we also have a backup style. Typically, this second style is dictated by our situation; the demands of our particular job if at work, the demands of domestic life if at home. We refer to the backup style as our "secondary style." Most people vacillate frequently between their primary and secondary styles. As a result, our overall or specific style becomes a combination of these two styles. It's like mixing lemon into tea: The concoction has a flavor all its own.

Here we know about one's unique flavor. For example, if the Profile revealed your primary style to be Director and your secondary style to be Harmonizer, then this creates an identifiable pattern of communicating called the Persuader. This style is highlighted below.

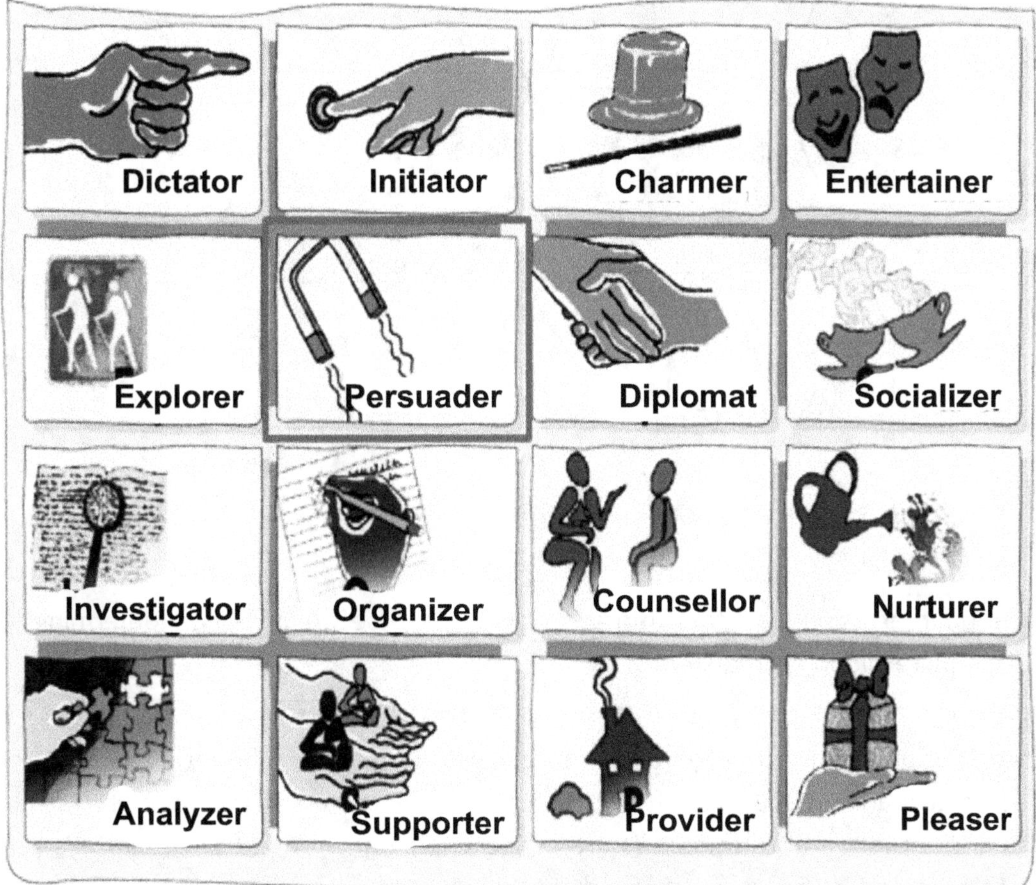

Fig. 5.2

The Matrix can be somewhat confusing at first, but it's a very useful tool once you understand how it works. In fact, once you instill in your mind a mental image of the Matrix, you can use it to identify another person's communication style, even if he or she hasn't taken the survey.

If you split the Matrix into equal quarters, or quadrants, then each quadrant illustrates a primary style; Director, Expresser, Thinker, or Harmonizer.

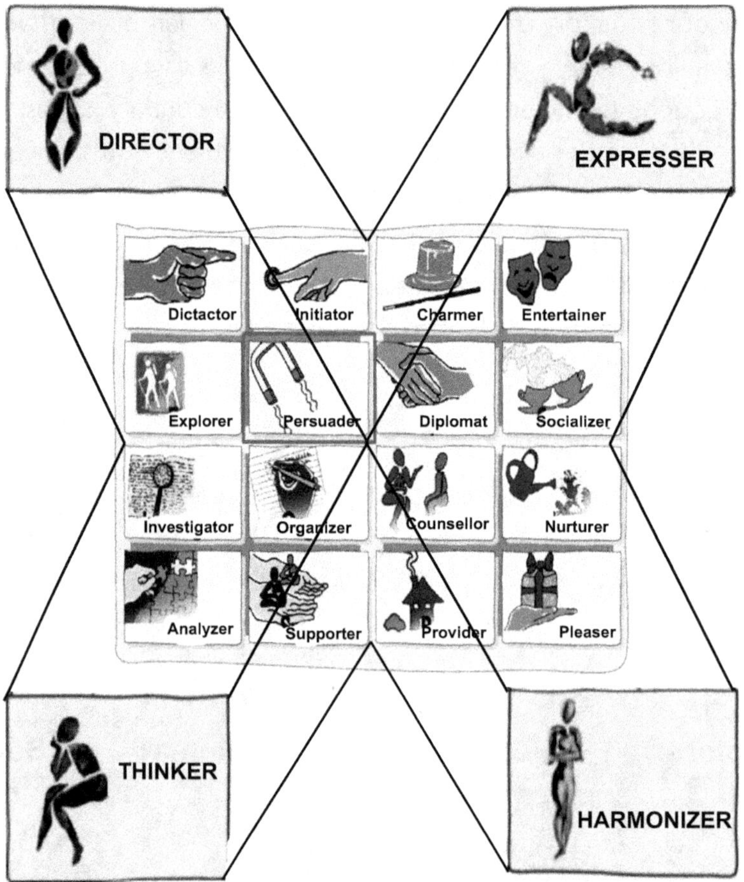

Fig. 5.3

Each quadrant contains four more squares. Your secondary style determines your particular square within each quadrant.

Here's how it works, using the Organizer as an example:

Step 1: Your primary style governs your placement in one of the four quadrants of the Matrix. Directors are in the upper left of the Matrix. Expressers are in the upper right. Thinkers are in the lower left, and Harmonizers are in the lower right. Since the Organizer's primary style is Thinker, he's in the lower-left quadrant.

Step 2: Once you've located your quadrant, cover up the other three. Pretend they don't exist. In this case, you would cover up the top half of the Matrix and the lower-right quadrant. The only quadrant visible would be the Thinker quadrant.

Step 3: The Thinker quadrant is divided into four smaller squares. Each has a label, like Investigator or Supporter. Use the same rule of thumb as the first step. If your secondary style is Director, then the upper-left square is your square (Investigator): if your secondary style is Expresser, then the upper-right square (Organizer) represents you.; if your secondary is also Thinker, then the lower-left square is yours (Analyzer); and if your secondary style is Harmonizer, then the lower-right square is yours (Supporter). In this case, the secondary style is Expresser, which makes this person an Organizer.

The Matrix is a very helpful tool because it lets you see the relationship between all sixteen styles at a glance. You can see how the styles at the top of the Matrix are the most assertive, while those at the bottom are the least so. How those on the left side are most analytical, while those on the right are the most intuitive. Take the survey!

Filters and Frames

The combined workings of filters and frames; both of which occur within our subconscious ; help us define the four basic styles of communicating. Some people set their filters so that more attention is placed on facts; some set them to allow more feelings to come through. Some people set their frames so that their responses are more assertive; some set their frames so that they respond with questions.

Using filters and frames, you can distill the four basic communication styles to these terms:

Directors: Filter for facts and respond assertively.

Expressers: Filter for feelings and respond assertively.

Thinkers: Filter for facts and respond by probing.

Harmonizers: Filter for feelings and respond by probing.

This is not to say that the only thing that distinguishes Directors from Expressers is that one filters for facts and the other for feelings. The behaviors of each communication style are more complex and varied than that. But certain behaviors are "markers" for each style, and these markers can help us identify a person's style. A marker is simply a specific behavior we look for in another person and in ourselves.

For example, one marker would be sensitivity to people's feelings. That's a clue that the person filters are set for feelings. A second marker is how often someone cites specific facts. A third marker is one's level of assertiveness. And a fourth marker is the extent to which one probes and inquires for more information. Each marker is a clue to help you determine a person's style. Understanding these markers is the first step to interpreting the styles of people around you.

Corner Styles

Some people; approximately one in a hundred are so-called "corner styles." The four corner styles are Director, Entertainer, Analyzer, and Pleaser. Corner styles occur when a person's score for one basic communication style is ten points higher than the score for any of the others. Corner styles have particular challenges to face in developing their communication skills. Because they don't regularly use a secondary, backup style, their communications tend to be less adaptable and flexible.

Blended Styles

Some people truly have two styles and occupy two places on the Matrix. We call these people "blended styles." A blended style occurs when a person's high score is identical for two of the basic communication styles. For example, a person who scores 35 for both Thinker and Director would be a blend of Investigator and Explorer.

If you have a blended style, don't worry. It's a perfectly natural out-growth of. Taking the survey again might slightly alter your score, and thus give you a neater fit within a particular square on the Matrix. But your score the first time you take the survey is typically the truest reflection of your style. And a person who has a blended style can get just as much out of Straight Talk as someone who occupies single square on the Matrix.

After you read the descriptions of each specific style, it may be readily evident which specific style is yours. If so, adopt it as your own. The purpose of the Matrix is to help you improve your communications, not to shoehorn you into a particular category or give you a label. As you begin to familiarize yourself with each style, certain themes begin to emerge about what constitutes a competent communicator. Once you start to appreciate the full spectrum of styles, you can also begin fitting your colleagues and friends into the Matrix. You can start to appreciate the dynamic shifts between communication styles. You can see how those styles at the top of the Matrix are the most assertive, while those at the bottom are the least assertive. How those on the left side are the most analytical, while those on the right are the most free flowing.

EXERCISE

1. What is communication style?
2. How many types of communication styles are there in a regular communication?
3. What is direct style of communication?
4. How direct style different from spirited style of communication?
5. How a person with considerate style may become popular ?
6. Describe 'the communication style matrix'.
7. Compare spirited style of communication with systematic style of communication.

Unit III

Chapter ... 6

BASIC LISTENING SKILLS

♦ **LEARNING OBJECTIVES** ♦

Objectives of this chapter are:

- *To make the learners understand the concept of self awareness.*
- *To make them able to differentiate between active and passive listening.*
- *To make them listen and understand the conversation even in difficult situations.*

6.1 INTRODUCTION

Listening skill is the ability to understand English when it is spoken. It is a receptive skill. It is the first skill that provides background to language learning. The student listens to oral speech in English, then separates into segments, the stretch of utterances he hears, groups them into words, phrases, and sentences, and, finally, he/she understands the message these carry. It is always there in every linguistic activity. Listening is important for casual chats, face-to-face encounters, and telephone messages, for enjoyment of radio and television programs, formal lectures, for understanding lectures, and many other activities. There is a need for an active involvement of the self for the efficient performance of listening.

Lundsteen (1979), "Listening is a complex, multi-step process by which spoken language is converted into meaning in the mind." Wolvin and Coakly (1985) have identified three steps in the process of listening which are receiving, attending and assigning meaning. In the first step, listeners receive the aural stimuli or the combined aural and visual stimuli presented by the speaker. In the second step, listeners focus on or attend to select stimuli while ignoring other distracting stimuli. In the third step, listeners assign meaning to or understand the speaker's message. Listening, thinking, and remembering go together. They are not separate acts a student may tend to focus on these as independent items. The teacher should organize her lesson and its presentation and teaching in the class in such a way that listening, thinking, and remembering are all integrated in listening comprehension.

(6.1)

Out of the four basic skills of English language, listening is the fundamental skill and is prerequisite to learn speaking. Through listening we get all information related to the world, it may be related with academic and economic purposes or just for entertainment.

Sub-skills of Listening: Rosts (1990) has distinguished following sub-skills of listening:

Perception is recognizing prominence within utterances, including discriminating sounds in words, especially phonemic contrasts, discriminating strong and weak forms, phonetic change, at word boundaries and identifying use of stress and pitch (information units, emphasis, etc.).

Interpretation is formulating content sense of utterance, conceptual framework and interpreting (possible) speaker intention. Content sense of utterance includes deducing the meaning of unfamiliar words and inferring implicit information. Formulating a conceptual framework linking utterances includes constructing a theme over a stretch of discourse and predicting content. Interpreting (possible) speaker intention includes identifying an interpersonal frame (speaker-to-hearer), establishing (in) consistencies, noting contradictions, inadequate information, ambiguities, differentiating between fact and opinion.

Enacting skills means making an appropriate response (based on the above) and it includes selecting key points for the current task and integrating information with that from other sources and providing appropriate feedback to the speaker.

Purpose of Listening:

Galvin (1985) has identified the following purposes of listening:

- **Listening for Appreciation:** It can increase our enjoyment through radio and TV programs. Close attention will enable us to increase our own use of language.
- **Listening for Information:** Through informative listening we can find answers to the problems, get directions, hear news of current interest and get the opinions of others. It provides food for conservation and examples for the expansion of ideas, speeches and letters and in other writings.
- **Selective Listening (selecting certain features at a time):** The technique of selective listening consists fundamentally in listening only to certain features at a time. One should listen for only one feature or set of features at a time. Then, one should listen successively to all the features of a language. The features of selective listening are: phonetic feature, vocabulary and grammar (morphology and syntax).
- **Extensive Listening (general idea):** Stories, rhymes, songs, television advertisement, poems, fairy tales and legends are given for extensive listening. Through extensive listening, plenty of opportunity is given to develop and exercise one's listening skill in a natural way.
- **Intensive Listening (for details):** If a teacher wants to train the listeners to have the ability for detailed comprehension of meaning and to get them to particular features of language such as vocabulary, grammar or pronunciation, they must train the listeners in intensive listening practice.

Aims of Teaching Listening Skill:

Listening skill is being taught to enable the students to:

- Discriminate between the basic sounds and phonological features of English including vowels, consonants, diphthongs, and consonant clusters.
- Discriminate between the basic patterns of word stress, sentence stress and intonation.
- Understand meaning of words, phrases and sentences in context.
- Understand statements, questions, instructions and commands.
- Respond to simple and complex oral instructions, requests and directions, conveyed in person or by telephone.
- Understand the main ideas and some significant details of simple spoken narratives and descriptive texts.
- Follow directions given orally.
- Grasp the substance and central idea of what is heard.
- Maintain his/her listening attention for a reasonable length of time.
- Listen to poems, songs, parodies, music and enjoy them.
- Listen with understanding discussions on different topics.

A skill listening may be taught for listening for sound perception and listening for comprehension. The first one is teaching for sound perception; here the students may have to be taught and exposed to discrimination of sounds used in English in isolation as well as in combination. These sounds are vowel and consonant sounds, their pronunciation and discrimination of similar sounds in words. It is usually practiced at early stages of listening. The second one is teaching how to listen a context, how to deduce meaning for an unfamiliar word, how to recognize theme over a discourse, the significance of pauses between words and phrases, sentence intonation etc. These two modes are important and inseparable for teaching of listening comprehension. Because the ultimate goal of listening is to listen for information so students listen to understand as part of using English for communication purposes.

Techniques of Developing Listening Skill

For developing listening skill we can use following techniques:

- **We may have exercises at the phonological level of English:** These will include the following: Aural discrimination exercises for segmental sounds, aural discrimination exercises for supra-segmental such as stress and intonation, stress placement exercises etc. Its examples are repetition of individual word or sentence by the children and crossing out of the sound written on the sheet, by listening that sound on tape.

- **We may also have listening comprehension exercises** which relate to listening in the process of reading a material. In these exercises, we may ask the students to number the words in the order in which they heard them, ask students to cross out what is not correct for the passage, ask students to identify the words with the sound specified, ask students to identify whether the words and phrases they heard in pairs are the same or different drills.

- **Dictation** is an excellent drill for developing listening comprehension.
- **Recoding exercises** in which you may ask the students to circle the sentence which has the same meaning as the one they hear may be given for listening comprehension practice.
- **Listen to the passage** and check all the appropriate answers.
- Use of a **cassette recorder**.
- **Listening for the message:** Read from a well-graded book or play a message on tape and ask students to say or write the essential parts of the message they just heard. Let the students concentrate on the general theme or the central message, instead of on specific words or phrases.
- **Responding with physical movement:** Instructions will be given orally and the listener has to act accordingly by making physical movements.
- **Making objects:** Oral instruction will be given by the teacher and listener has to follow it. For example – how to make a kite from a paper, coloring the pictures.
- **Tick off items:** The students listen to the text and tick the required items which appear on the work sheet.
- **Grids:** The teacher reads out the information and the pupils have to fill the grids.
- **Family Tree:** This can be drawn on the blackboard for the learners to copy down. The learners listen to the teacher or the tape and fill in whatever is asked for in the task.
- **Bio-data forms, bank or passport forms, railway reservation forms, timetables** can all be used as grids. There could be conversation between two persons on a tape. Let the learners fill in the details in the blanks after listening to the tape.
- **Flow chart:** Flow charts can be used as task sheet for listening activity. For example, the learners listen to a tape or teacher's instructions on how to make a tea and fill in the blanks in the chart.
- **Using maps:** Maps can be used as task sheets in the listening activities to (a) Mark a route, (b) Locate a particular place, (c) Locate where different places are and different people live.
- **Predictions:** In this activity, the students are told an incident or a story with various possible climaxes. They listen to the full or part of the narrative and try to predict the later part.
- **Summarizing:** The students listen to the text and understand the important facts and events and summarize them in brief.

- In **Problem solving listening comprehension** exercises, students listen to the description or presentation of a problem and solve it, by doing what is required of them.

6.2 SELF-AWARENESS

Self-awareness is having a clear perception of your personality, including strengths, weaknesses, thoughts, beliefs, motivation, and emotions. Self-awareness allows you to understand other people, how they perceive you, your attitude and your responses to them in the moment. We might quickly assume that we are self aware, but it is helpful to have a relative scale for awareness. If you have ever been in an auto accident you may have experienced everything happening in slow motion and noticed details of your thought process and the event. This is a state of heightened awareness. With practice we can learn to engage these types of heightened states and see new opportunities for interpretations in our thoughts, emotions, and conversations. Having awareness creates the opportunity to make changes in behaviour and beliefs.

1. **Why Develop Self-awareness:** As you develop self-awareness you are able to make changes in the thoughts and interpretations you make in your mind. Changing the interpretations in your mind allows you to change your emotions. Self-awareness is one of the attributes of Emotional Intelligence and an important factor in achieving success. Self-awareness is the first step in creating what you want and mastering your life. Where you focus, your attention, your emotions, reactions, personality and behaviour determine where you go in life. Having self-awareness allows you to see where your thoughts and emotions are taking you. It also allows you to take control of your emotions, behaviour, and personality so you can make changes you want. Until you are aware in the moment of your thoughts, emotions, words, and behaviour, you will have difficulty making changes in the direction of your life.

2. **Self-awareness in Relationships:** Relationships are easy until there is emotional turmoil. This is the same whether you are at work or in your personal life. When you can change the interpretation in your mind of what you think you can change your emotions and shift the emotional quality of your relationships. When you can change the emotions in your relationships you open up entirely new possibilities in your life. Having a clear understanding of your thought and behaviour patterns helps you understand other people. This ability to empathize facilitates better personal and professional relationships.

3. **Develop Self-awareness:** Self-awareness is developed through practices in focusing your attention on the details of your personality and behaviour. It isn't learned from reading a book. When you read a book you are focusing your attention on the conceptual ideas in the book. You can develop an intellectual understanding of the ideas of self-awareness from a book, but this is not the same. With your attention in a book you are practicing and not paying attention to your own behaviour, emotions and personality.

Think of learning to be mindful and self-aware as learning to dance. When learning to dance we have to pay attention to how and where our feet move, our hands and body motion, what our partner is doing, music, beat, floor space, and other dancers. Dancing isn't learned from books and self-awareness isn't either. A dancer needs awareness of their body movements. Self-awareness is what you develop when you pay attention to your expressions of thought, emotions, and behaviour.

If you have an emotional reaction of anger or frustration, you notice many of the thoughts and small triggers that build up towards those emotions. You also notice moments when you can change the interpretations in your mind, or not believe what you are thinking. In this heightened awareness you instinctively make better choices in your thought process long before an emotional reaction or destructive behaviour.

Making changes in your behaviour is much easier to do when you catch them early in the dynamic, before the momentum of thought and emotion has gathered steam. The changes in your mind and behaviour become simple and easy steps when you develop self-awareness.

To increase your awareness the first step is to practice becoming the observer. Developing self-awareness is a great way of learning more about yourself and what you're capable of. Self-awareness is really just about being aware of who we are. It can relate to knowing your own values, your beliefs, personal preferences and tendencies. Because we are all different in the way we react to things, it can be really helpful to start thinking about how we work best, including things like: how we learn best, our talents and abilities, personality traits, political beliefs, values.

You know how famous people always say "Stay true to yourself". This is actually a really important advice, but it's not easy to stay true to yourself if you don't know who you are. By becoming self-aware and understanding your strengths and limitations, you open up opportunities that just aren't available if you don't know yourself.

How to work on itself-awareness

- **Assess your self-talk:** The first step in self-awareness is to listen to yourself. What's going on in your mind? Is it a series of negative thoughts that make you feel pretty crap? Or are you always looking on the bright side?

  In practice: Take a couple of minutes each day to just sit in silence and listen to what you're thinking. One way of getting your inner voice going is to stand in front of a mirror and hear what you're saying to yourself about how you look. It might even help to write down your thoughts so you can get a better idea of how positive or negative they are.

- **Use your senses:** Our senses (sight and sound in particular) provide us with a huge insight into the world, ourselves, other people and situations. But these senses are often viewed through a filter of our own self talk. For example, a frown does not always mean someone's angry and someone groaning doesn't mean you're boring. When our mind is determining how we see things it can be easy to start feeling hurt.

  In practice: Next time you feel like someone is judging you or has made you feel bad about yourself, take a step back and write down why you think this. Ask yourself, could these actions have been interpreted differently? You might actually find that your interpretation was clouded by your own negative thoughts.

- **Get your feelings out:** This can be hard if you're not the kind of person who likes to think too deeply about your feelings, but it can be really worthwhile. Our feelings are spontaneous and emotional responses to the things we experience. Like our senses, they give us good information about what's going on around us. Sometimes it can be hard to tune into feelings, but there are a couple of physical signs that you can look for which might help. Some examples include: A warm feeling in your face might mean you're embarrassed; a feeling of 'butterflies' in your tummy can mean you're nervous; clenching your teeth might mean you're angry.

  In practice: Look out for physical signs which might indicate how you're feeling. By engaging with how you're feeling, you can get a better insight into what you like, what makes you uncomfortable and what makes you angry.

6.3 ACTIVE LISTENING

Listening is the most fundamental component of interpersonal communication skills. Listening is not something that just happens (that is hearing); listening is an active process in which a conscious decision is made to listen to and understand the messages of the speaker. Listeners should not be tempted to jump in with questions or comments every time there are a few seconds of silence. Active listening involves giving the other person time to explore their thoughts and feelings, they should, therefore, be given adequate time for that.

Like critical thinking and problem-solving, active listening is a soft skill that is held in high regard by employers. When interviewing for jobs, use active listening techniques to show the interviewer the interpersonal skills you have in drawing people out. Active listening can also significantly reduce the nervousness you might be feeling during an interview because it redirects your focus from what is going on inside of your head to what the needs of your perspective employer are. By placing your focus, through active listening, squarely upon the interviewer, you prove that you are interested in the organization's challenges and successes; are ready to help them problem-solve work issues; and are a team player as opposed to being a self-absorbed job candidate. Active listening is a communication technique used in counseling, training, and conflict resolution. It requires that the listener fully concentrate, understand, respond and then remember what is being said. This is opposed to reflective listening where the listener repeats back to the speaker what they have just heard to confirm understanding of both parties.

Active listening is the process by which an individual secures information from another individual or group. The 'active' element involves taking steps to draw out information that might not otherwise be shared. Even if you yourself are the person being interviewed for a job, think of 'active' listening as being your golden opportunity to 'interview' and build rapport with your interviewer. Active listening is a skill that can be acquired and developed with practice. However, active listening can be difficult to master and will, therefore, take time and patience to develop. 'Active listening' means, as its name suggests, actively listening.

That is fully concentrating on what is being said rather than just passively 'hearing' the message of the speaker. Active listening involves listening with all senses. As well as giving full attention to the speaker, it is important that the 'active listener' is also 'seen' to be listening – otherwise the speaker may conclude that what they are talking about is uninteresting to the listener.

Active listening not only means focusing fully on the speaker but also actively showing verbal and non-verbal signs of listening. Generally speakers want listeners to demonstrate 'active listening' by responding appropriately to what they are saying. Appropriate responses to listening can be both verbal and non-verbal.

Signs of Active Listening

Non-verbal signs of attentive or active listening are more likely to display at least some of these signs. However these signs may not be appropriate in all situations and across all cultures.

- **Smile:** Small smiles can be used to show that the listener is paying attention to what is being said or as a way of agreeing or being happy about the messages being received. Combined with nods of the head, smiles can be powerful in affirming that messages are being listened to and understood.

- **Eye Contact:** It is normal and usually encouraging for the listener to look at the speaker. Eye contact can however be intimidating, especially for more shy speakers – gauge how much eye contact is appropriate for any given situation. Combine eye contact with smiles and other non-verbal messages to encourage the speaker.

- **Posture:** Posture can tell a lot about the sender and receiver in interpersonal interactions. The attentive listener tends to lean slightly forward or sideways whilst sitting. Other signs of active listening may include a slight slant of the head or resting the head on one hand.

- **Mirroring:** Automatic reflection/mirroring of any facial expressions used by the speaker can be a sign of attentive listening. These reflective expressions can help to show sympathy and empathy in more emotional situations. Attempting to consciously mimic facial expressions (that is, not automatic reflection of expressions) can be a sign of inattention.

- **Distraction:** The active listener will not be distracted and therefore will refrain from fidgeting, looking at a clock or watch, doodling, playing with their hair or picking their fingernails.

6.4 BECOMING AN ACTIVE LISTENER

We all go through our daily lives engaging in many conversations with friends, co-workers, and our family members. But most of the time, we don't listen as well as we could or sometimes should. We're often distracted by other things in the environment, such as the television, the internet, our cell phones, or something else. We think we're listening to the other person, but we're really not giving them our full attention. Active listening is all about building rapport, understanding, and trust. By learning this skill, you will become a better listener and actually hear what the other person is saying—not just what you think they are saying or what you want to hear. It also helps a person feel free to continue talking even if the person they are talking to doesn't have a lot to offer the other person (other than their ear). It takes a lot of concentration and determination to be an active listener. Old habits are hard to break, and if your listening skills are as bad as many people's are, then there's a lot of habit-breaking to do. Start using active listening techniques today to become a better communicator, improve your workplace productivity, and develop better relationships.

There are following key active listening techniques. They all help you ensure that you hear the other person and that the other person knows you are hearing what they say.

- **Pay attention but be relaxed:** Now that you've made eye contact, relax. You don't have to stare fixedly at the other person. You can look away now and then and carry on like a normal person. The important thing is to be attentive. The dictionary says that to "attend" another person means to be present and remain ready to serve. Mentally screen out distractions, like background activity and noise. In addition, try not to focus on the speaker's accent or speech mannerisms to the point where they become distractions. Finally, don't be distracted by your own thoughts, feelings, or biases.

Give the speaker your undivided attention, and acknowledge the message. Recognize that non-verbal communication also "speaks" loudly.

- Look at the speaker directly.
- Put aside distracting thoughts.
- Don't mentally prepare a rebuttal!
- Avoid being distracted by environmental factors, for example, side conversations.
- Listen to the speaker's body language.

Show that you're listening:
- Use your own body language and gestures to convey your attention.
- Nod occasionally.
- Smile and use other facial expressions.
- Note your posture and make sure it is open and inviting.
- Encourage the speaker to continue with small verbal comments like 'yes' and 'uh huh'.

Provide feedback:
- Our personal filters, assumptions, judgments, and beliefs can distort what we hear. As a listener, your role is to understand what is being said. This may require you to reflect what is being said and ask questions.
- Reflect what has been said by paraphrasing. "What I'm hearing is," and "Sounds like you are saying," are great ways to reflect back.
- Ask questions to clarify certain points. "What do you mean when you say," "Is this what you mean?"

- Summarize the speaker's comments periodically.
- If you find yourself responding emotionally to what someone said, say so, and ask for more information: "I may not understand you correctly and I find myself taking what you said personally".

Defer judgement:

- Interrupting is a waste of time. It frustrates the speaker and limits full understanding of the message.
- Allow the speaker to finish each point before asking questions.
- Don't interrupt with counter arguments.

Respond appropriately:

- Active listening is a model for respect and understanding. You are gaining information and perspective. You add nothing by attacking the speaker or otherwise putting him or her down.
- Be candid, open, and honest in your response.
- Assert your opinions respectfully.
- Treat the other person in a way that you think he or she would want to be treated.

Restating:

- To show you are listening, repeat every so often what you think the person said, not by parroting, but by paraphrasing what you heard in your own words. For example, "Let's see if I'm clear about this. . ."

Summarizing:

- Bring together the facts and pieces of the problem to check understanding for example, "So it sounds to me as if . . ." Or, "Is that it?"

Minimal encouragers:

- Use brief, positive prompts to keep the conversation going and show you are listening; for example, "umm-hmmm," "Oh?" "I understand," "Then?" "And?"

Reflecting:

- Instead of just repeating, reflect the speaker's words in terms of feelings; for example, "This seems really important to you. . ."

Emotion labeling:

- Putting feelings into words will often help a person to see things more objectively. To help the person begin, use "door openers" for example, "I'm sensing that you're feeling frustrated... worried... anxious..."

Probing:

- Ask questions to draw the person out and get deeper and more meaningful information; for example, "What do you think would happen if you...?"

Validation:

- Acknowledge the individual's problems, issues, and feelings. Listen openly and with empathy, and respond in an interested way; for example, "I appreciate your willingness to talk about such a difficult issue..."

Effective pause:

- Deliberately pause at key points for emphasis. This will tell the person you are saying something that is very important to them.

Silence:

- Allow for comfortable silences to slow down the exchange. Give a person time to think as well as talk. Silence can also be very helpful in diffusing an unproductive interaction.

"I" messages:

- By using "I" in your statements, you focus on the problem, not the person. An I-message lets the person know what you feel and why; for example, "I know you have a lot to say, but I need to..."

Redirecting:

- If someone is showing signs of being overly aggressive, agitated, or angry, this is the time to shift the discussion to another topic.

Consequences:

- Part of the feedback may involve talking about the possible consequences of inaction. Take your cues from what the person is saying; for example, "What happened the last time you stopped taking the medicine your doctor prescribed?"

Face the Speaker and Maintain Eye Contact:

Talking to someone while they scan the room, study a computer screen, or gaze out the window is like trying to hit a moving target. How much of the person's divided attention you are actually getting? Fifty percent? Five percent? If the person were your child you might demand, "Look at me when I'm talking to you," but that's not the sort of thing we say to a friend or colleague. In most Western cultures, eye contact is considered a basic ingredient of effective communication. When we talk, we look each other in the eye. That doesn't mean that you can't carry on a conversation from across the room, or from another room, but if the conversation continues for any length of time, you (or the other person) will get up and move. The desire for better communication pulls you together. Do your conversational partners the courtesy of turning to face them. Put aside papers, books, the phone and other distractions. Look at them, even if they don't look at you. Shyness, uncertainty, shame, guilt, or other emotions, along with cultural taboos, can inhibit eye contact in some people under some circumstances.

Keep an open mind:

Listen without judging the other person or mentally criticizing the things she tells you. If what she says alarms you, go ahead and feel alarmed, but don't say to yourself, "Well, that was a stupid move." As soon as you indulge in judgmental bemusements, you've compromised your effectiveness as a listener.

Listen without jumping to conclusions:

Remember that the speaker is using language to represent the thoughts and feelings inside her brain. You don't know what those thoughts and feelings are and the only way you'll find out is by listening.

Don't be a sentence-grabber:

Occasionally my partner can't slow his mental pace enough to listen effectively, so he tries to speed up mine by interrupting and finishing my sentences. This usually lands him way off base, because he is following his own train of thought and doesn't learn where my thoughts are headed. After a couple of rounds of this, I usually ask, "Do you want to have this conversation by yourself, or do you want to hear what I have to say?" I wouldn't do that with everyone, but it works with him.

Listen to the words and try to picture what the speaker is saying:

Allow your mind to create a mental model of the information being communicated. Whether a literal picture, or an arrangement of abstract concepts, your brain will do the necessary work if you stay focused, with senses fully alert. When listening for long stretches, concentrate on, and remember, key words and phrases. When it's your turn to listen, don't spend the time planning what to say next. You can't rehearse and listen at the same time. Think only about what the other person is saying. Finally, concentrate on what is being said, even if it bores you. If your thoughts start to wander, immediately force yourself to refocus.

Don't interrupt and don't impose your "solutions":

Children used to be taught that it's rude to interrupt. I'm not sure that message is getting across anymore. Certainly the opposite is being modeled on the majority of talk shows and reality programs, where loud, aggressive, in-your-face behaviour is condoned, if not encouraged. We all think and speak at different rates. If you are a quick thinker and an agile talker, the burden is only how to relax your pace for the slower, more thoughtful communicator—or for the guy who has trouble expressing himself.

When listening to someone talk about a problem, refrain from suggesting solutions:

Most of us don't want your advice anyway. If we do, we'll ask for it. Most of us prefer to figure out our own solutions. We need you to listen and help us do that. Somewhere way down the line, if you are absolutely bursting with a brilliant solution, at least get the speaker's permission. Ask, "Would you like to hear my ideas?"

Wait for the speaker to pause to ask clarifying questions:

When you don't understand something, of course you should ask the speaker to explain it to you. But rather than interrupt, wait until the speaker pauses. Then say something like, "Back up a second. I didn't understand what you just said about..."

Ask questions only to ensure understanding:

At lunch, a colleague is excitedly telling you about her trip to Vishakhapatnam and all the wonderful things she did and saw. In the course of this chronicle, she mentions that she spent some time with a mutual friend. You jump in with, "Oh, I haven't heard from Alka in ages. How is she?" and, just like that, the discussion shifts to Alka and her life. This particular conversational affront happens all the time. Our questions lead people in directions that have nothing to do with where they thought they were going. Sometimes we work our way back to the original topic, but very often we don't.

Try to feel what the speaker is feeling:

If you feel sad when the person with whom you are talking expresses sadness, joyful when she expresses joy, fearful when she describes her fears and convey those feelings through your facial expressions and words then your effectiveness as a listener is assured. Empathy is the heart and soul of good listening.

To experience empathy, you have to put yourself in the other person's place and allow yourself to feel what it is like to be her at that moment. This is not an easy thing to do. It takes energy and concentration. But it is a generous and helpful thing to do, and it facilitates communication like nothing else does.

Give the speaker regular feedback:

Show that you understand where the speaker is coming from by reflecting the speaker's feelings. "You must be thrilled!" "What a terrible ordeal for you." "I can see that you are confused." If the speaker's feelings are hidden or unclear, then occasionally paraphrase the content of the message. Or just nod and show your understanding through appropriate facial expressions and an occasional well-timed "hmmm" or "uh huh." The idea is to give the speaker some proof that you are listening, and that you are following her train of thought—not off indulging in your own fantasies while she talks to the ether. In task situations, regardless of whether at work or home, always restate instructions and messages to be sure you understand correctly.

Pay attention to what isn't said; to nonverbal cues:

If you exclude email, the majority of direct communication is probably nonverbal. We glean a great deal of information about each other without saying a word. Even over the telephone, you can learn almost as much about a person from the tone and cadence of her voice than from anything she says. When I talk to my best friend, it doesn't matter what we chat about, if I hear a lilt and laughter in her voice, I feel reassured that she's doing well.

Face to face with a person, you can detect enthusiasm, boredom, or irritation very quickly in the expression around the eyes, the set of the mouth, the slope of the shoulders. These are clues you can't ignore. When listening, remember that words convey only a fraction of the message.

In conversations that result in agreements about future obligations or activities, summarizing will not only ensure accurate follow-through, it will feel perfectly natural. In conversations that do not include agreements, if summarizing feels awkward just explain that you are doing it as an exercise.

6.5 LISTENING IN DIFFICULT SITUATIONS

Difficult listening situations don't mean that you have to hear poorly. With these tips you may be able to improve your hearing and listening skills regardless of the intruding sounds. What's a Difficult Listening Situation? Do any of these sound familiar to you?

- Dinner at a restaurant, where it seems like you can hear the table next to you more than your own table?

- Talking with someone who keeps covering their mouth?
- Trying to talk with someone on the other side of the room?
- Listening to a lecturer who is standing far away from you?
- Someone talking really fast, or really loud?

If you have difficulty in hearing in situations like these, that's normal. There are easy ways that you can make the best of a difficult listening environment, and work to improve your speech understanding and comprehension skills.

The first step in working to improve your hearing is getting hearing people to understand your needs as a person with hearing loss. Most people won't mind doing certain things to help you hear better, but it's up to you to tell them what these things are.

General Tips to Improve Your Hearing

- Ask them to speak clearly and naturally, but to not shout or exaggerate their pronunciation. Speaking slowly helps to improve comprehension a lot.
- If you don't understand it the first time, just ask them to repeat or rephrase what they said.
- Ask them to move closer to you, or you can move closer to them.
- If you can't see their face or gestures because it's too dark, ask to move to an area with good lighting.
- If someone is eating, or covering their face while talking to you, just ask them to stop while they're talking.
- If you're in a noisy situation, like a room where a TV is turned on in the background, move to another room if possible.
- If there's a loud noise that you know will be over soon, like having a loud truck drive by, just wait for it to end and then get back to your conversation.
- If the information is important, like directions to somewhere specific, ask to have them written down as well.
- Concentration is important but tiring. Don't be afraid of taking regular breaks, and if you return to a group conversation just ask someone to sum up the main parts of what was said while you were away.
- When out at an event like a movie or at church arrive early to make sure you get an optimal seat, one that is close to the speaker, but far away from walls.
- If you're going to a movie or the theater, read reviews in advance to familiarize yourself with the plot.
- Instead of stressing out by focusing on hearing every single word, try to understand the bigger picture. Use verbal and non-verbal cues to get a sense of what the speaker means instead of what they're saying.
- Ask the venue in advance if they can make sure the speaker has a microphone.
- If you use hearing aids or a cochlear implant ask the venue if they have assistive listening devices in place like an FM system or loop induction system.

For hearing aid users, some listening situations are more problematic than others. Listening in noisy surroundings, for example, is often more problematic than listening in quiet situations. Often the ability to focus on specific sounds is reduced when you have a hearing loss. Everyday sounds such as noise from a dishwasher or many people talking at the same time can easily become disturbing background sounds.

Everyday sounds can be disturbing: Normally, we associate being at home with relaxation and quiet surroundings. For people with normal hearing, most household sounds are insignificant. But for those with a hearing loss, everyday sounds such as those from a dishwasher, water dripping or noise from a vacuum cleaner can be very disturbing.

TV and radio sounds become background noise: Otherwise pleasant sounds can be disturbing if heard at the same time. Sounds from the radio or television are appreciated on their own, but if mixed together with people talking they can become disturbing too.

Experiencing music: Hearing aid users experience the quality of music, whether live or recorded, in very different ways. Some find that music heard through a hearing aid sounds natural, while others find that it differs too much from the way they expect it to sound. Situations where anyone may feel difficulty in listening are described below:

Television: Hearing the television is probably one of the most important issues for those who are hard of hearing. Between husbands and wives and partners and family members arguments are prone to occur – too loud versus not loud enough. Television viewing should be relaxing for all concerned and never the source of contention. There is no need for TV martyrs. Sound levels can be adapted to those watching on an individual basis. It is just a matter of setting it up. For those who lost hearing ability they can enjoy watching the television, having different programs with subtitles.

The clarity of sound heard from the TV is not dependent on the volume. Simply turning up the sound helps only very slightly and sometimes not at all. This is because the clarity depends on the distance between the loud speaker on the TV set and the receiver of the hearing aid. The echo of the sound within the room distorts the clarity. Much greater clarity is obtained if the sound receiver is in the form of a listening device and is very close to the TV set. The sound is then received close to the source and transmitted by radio direct to the receiver (worn by the person with hearing loss). This avoids any echo.

Loop systems can be used. These involve either an individual telecoil loop (similar to those in public places) or a room loop where a wire encircles the whole room so that all those within the area of the loop benefit – hearing aids need to be switched to the T position.

Headphones for individual use are another method of hearing. They can be wired or alternatively wirelessly linked to the TV. The wireless link to the TV is ideal. Headphones can be worn over a hearing aid.

In the car: Background noise prevents hearing of general conversation in the car but a wireless linked listener can be used – this can be hand held and passed to the person who is talking. In some cars use of the telecoil can result in an electronic hum. This is caused by the telecoil and not by the listening device. The hum can be a nuisance. It is well worth knowing that use can be made of a wireless linked listener to listen to the radio whilst travelling. If the microphone is placed very close to the speaker, the sound from the speaker drowns out much of the background wind and traffic noise. Use can be made of this when travelling alone. In my car the loud speaker is near the floor and so the microphone is best placed attached to leg – even tucked into a sock. This is then very effective for listening to the news programs.

Headphones linked to a radio might be tried, but these should not be so efficient as to cut out the sound of car horns, ambulance sirens etc.

Social gatherings, restaurants and pubs: Radio listeners are the only way. In a one-to-one situation the transmitting microphone is placed in the best place to hear the conversation. This might be around the neck of one's companion or in a strategic place on the table. The receiver is on a neck loop worn by the listener (telecoil setting on the HA is needed) or by means of an ear level receiver. They are highly effective. When two or more people are gathered the transmitting microphone can be placed on the table in the middle of the group. If background noise is present there may be problems – as there are even for those who have 'normal' hearing.

When talking in a one-to-one situation one can use the transmitting microphone, hand held, close to the mouth of the person to whom one is talking. This can be helpful.

The choice of a carpeted or well-furnished room is best and one should ideally sit with one's back to the wall. A directional microphone is useful directed away from unwanted sound sources.

If there is an area well away from music then that would make the best choice for a table. Obviously avoid sitting near any music loud speaker.

Attending lectures / meetings: Radio listeners are the only way. The speaker at a meeting is asked to wear the transmitting microphone. The listener can then sit at the back of the room. This is highly effective. In committee meeting the microphone is placed near the committee. This can then be effective but hearing comments from those distant is difficult.

Door bells, wake-up and fire alarms: To neglect to have fitted a fire alarm which is appropriate for your hearing loss is highly mistaken. Fire alarms save lives. If you are very hard of hearing it is wise to have an alarm which wakes you at night by vibrating. There are door bells which are connected to a vibrating signal which one wears.

EXERCISE

1. What is listening?
2. What is the difference between listening and hearing?
3. Highlight the importance of listening in daily interaction.
4. Why is self-awareness considered as important factor to enhance your personality?
5. How could you develop self-awareness?
6. Justify this statement with examples, "Listening skill is the most important skill to develop speaking skill, even then it is not taught separately to all Indian students".
7. What is active listening?
8. How is active listening different from passive listening?
9. Describe how to become an active listener.
10. How could you manage to listen in difficult situations?

Chapter ... 7

EFFECTIVE WRITTEN COMMUNICATION

♦ LEARNING OBJECTIVES ♦

Objectives of this chapter are:

- *To make the students understand the concept of effective writing.*
- *To make them able to use different words according to the context.*
- *To organise their message correctly.*

7.1 INTRODUCTION

Writing skill is the ability to write English correctly. Writing is a productive skill and it involves producing language rather than receiving it. Writing skills are specific abilities which help writers put their thoughts into words in a meaningful form and to mentally interact with the message. Writing skills can be ticket to better grades and greater academic achievement. Writing skills help the learner gain independence, comprehensibility, fluency and creativity in writing. It provides a relatively permanent record of information, opinions, beliefs, feelings, arguments, explanations, theories etc. Writing is an individual effort or work. It is a conscious, deliberate and planned activity. Writing allows us to share our communication not only with our contemporaries, but also with future generations.

According to **Billow (1981)**,"writing is a kind of 'magic'." Here magic means the process of transforming the abstract sounds into concrete scripts.

Writing is a form of encoded symbols in the form of print or impression. Writing more particularly, refers to two things: Writing as a noun, the thing that is written and writing as a verb, which designates the activity of writing. **Topkins** and **Hoskisson** (1995) provide five stages of writing process. They are: prewriting, drafting, revising, editing and presentation. **Prewriting** is the stage of getting-ready-to-write. In this stage, the student chooses a topic and organizes ideas for writing. The second stage, **drafting** stage is the time to pour out ideas with little concern about spelling, punctuation and other mechanical error. The third one is **revision** stage; in this stage, the writer refines ideas in his compositions. Activities in this stage are reading the rough draft, sharing the rough draft in a writing group and revising on the basis of feed-back. Next, the **editing** stage is the state of putting the piece of writing into its final form. The writer moves through three activities in this editing stage: getting distance from the composition, proof reading to locate the errors and correcting errors. Now the final draft is ready. In this stage, a young writer shares his compositions/writings with the real audience of classmates, other students, teachers and the parents.

Writing is one of the two expressive skills in the field of language learning, the other one being speaking. The correct messages, feelings, thoughts and experiences can only be communicated in written form. Writing aims at clear and efficient communication. Writing trains our eyes, ears and also develops our memory. Referring to the importance of writing, **Lord Bacon** says, "Reading makes a full man, conference a ready man and writing an exact man". What he means is that writing is a useful means of organizing thoughts and giving a precision. It is the practical side of language learning.

7.2 SUB-SKILLS OF WRITING SKILL

The writing skill includes a number of sub-skills. According to **Sobana** (2003), the sub-skills of writing skill are;

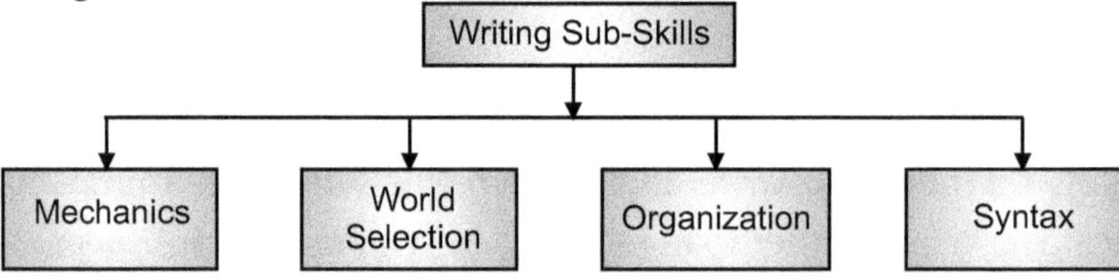

Fig. 7.1

(i)   **Mechanics**, which includes handwriting, spelling and punctuation.
(ii) **Word Selection**, which includes vocabulary, idioms and phrases.
(iii) **Organization**, which includes paragraphs, topic and cohesion.
(iv) **Syntax**, which includes sentence structure according to different grammatical rules.

In today's world of rapid-fast communication via texts and emails, most of us would rather shoot off a written message than make a phone call. It's fast, efficient when used properly, and it provides a nice document trail for our work records. Written communication is more important than ever, yet very few people know when writing is the right-or wrong – form of communication and fewer still can write well. Of course, like all other communication skills, good writing skills can be learned.

7.3 WHEN AND WHEN NOT TO USE WRITTEN COMMUNICATION

Sure, sending an email is easy. How many of us haven't written one while on hold with another call or in those few moments between one meeting and the next ? Texts are never easier and let you send information from virtually any where.

Yet when is written communication most effective, and when is it not ? There are a number of factors that can help you make that choice.

Complexity of the topic: Using written communication is an excellent choice for sharing information that is easily organized and easily understood by the independent reader. This means that the reader can read the communication and get the message clearly without additional information from you or other sources. Meeting, notices, answers to quick questions or quick clarifications are all easy to complete with written communication.

> Highly complex topics or lengthy explanations are not good choices for normal written communication. Written communication should 'stand alone' for the reader.

However, there is a point at which written communication becomes inefficient for one of several reasons. The information may be too complex to organize in a manner that will be intelligible to your reader without further assistance. The amount of explanation required to make the information intelligible might be cumbersome, leading to misinterpretation or lack of understanding. In the long run, you'll end up answering so many follow-up emails or phone calls that in these cases you would have been off having a face-to-face meeting or in a formal training session.

Amount of discussion required: If the topic is complex or involved enough that there will need to be a long exchange of discussion type emails, the longer you allow the exchange to continue in writing, the more you are risking that someone will misunderstand. Furthermore, you can't be assured that everyone who received the email has actually had the chance to participate in the discussion unless you are able to track the receipt of others' emails or require everyone to respond one way or the other. Therefore, decision making, long involved explanations or conversations, or controversial subjects are not usually good topics for written communication.

> Lengthy discussions by written communication (email) are not efficient, and each exchange risks meaning getting lost.

Shades of Meaning: We have learned from previous information that non verbal communication is the most important form of communication in getting your message delivered. When you are writing, you are left to the small portion of communication that is possible through words alone in getting your message through to your reader. So the more intense the emotions around a topic or the more important the message is, the less likely writing will be a successful form of communicating.

> Written communication alone does not allow for non-verbal communication-the most important aspect of getting your meaning across.

For example, it can be difficult to convey tone of voice, humor, sarcasm, or other shades of meaning in writing alone. Don't risk offending someone or causing confusion by someone not understanding your true meaning by trusting written communication with the task of conveying highly emotional or important information.

Formal communication: Although there are exceptions, written communication is still the common choice when the level of formality between two parties is high. For example, think about your customers or clients. Chances are that formal communication such as contract terms, sales agreement, account information, or other legal or administrative information will be transmitted in written form. This gives you both the information in a format that you can pass on as needed and gives you both reference material to help you in continuing your communication. As the level of formality decreases in the relationship, you are more likely to move from paper documentation to email documentation as well.

> The higher the level of formality of communication, the more likely you will use written communication and you will usually employ email more are the level of formality decreases.

7.4 WRITING EFFECTIVELY

Although some of the following information relates to either email or paper communication, it is mainly geared towards email since so much of our work involves email. However, you can apply most of the advice to paper communication as well.

Subject lines: When you are writing a letter or an email, the subject line of the communication is like the headline in a newspaper. It calls your attention to the communication and should also let you know what it is about. The best subject lines will also tell you what needs to be done-and will let the recipient prioritize which emails to open first and which ones to ignore for later or altogether.

What do these subject lines tell you about the information that will follow?
- Response to your email
- Question
- Hello
- Meeting
- Information for you

By these subject lines, can you tell any information about what will follow? Sure, the first one could be clear if the receiver has only written one email that day. But most of us handle dozens, if not hundreds of emails every week. It's unlikely the receiver will remember exactly what you are responding to.

The other subject lines are too general. They don't specify what information will be contained or what action the recipient needs to take. If there is important or urgent information included, it might go unread-or opened, scanned and dismissed.

Instead, try subject lines such as:
- Information on Open House Thursday, July 19, 2017-Please RSVP.
- Question Regarding the Change in Health Benefits-Response Needed.
- Meeting Regarding NBA Accreditation – Please Confirm Availability.
- Response to Your Question on the Marketing Plan for 2nd Quarter.

Each of these tells the reader what information they will find when they open the email, and also tells them whether or not they need to take action. The reader can decide which of these is most important and process the incoming emails in the best order.

Put the main points first: When you write your communication, you need to know exactly what, why and to whom you are writing. Are you simply giving information, asking for information or requesting the other person to take an action? If you can't narrow down the point, you either aren't ready to write or writing isn't the right choice of communication formats to use.

Once you know what the main point of your email is, you should put that first in the communication. We all tend to scan written communication to save time, focusing more at the top of the information than the bottom. Putting your main information at the top of the communication pulls the reader's attention to the main topic, request or instruction. You can follow with background information after you've stated the reason for writing - but if you start with background information, you risk your reader missing the point of the communication.

Here is a bad example:

Dear Vedant,

I spent some time with Divyanshi this morning reviewing the numbers from last quarter's sales results. I was concerned to see that there seems to be a downward trend in sales of the AquaRain, which is significantly different from what we forecasted. I am concerned that this might have an impact on our launch of the AquaRain Super planned for next quarter. I think we should meet with the marketing team and the sales team to see if we can identify any possible issues with the sales and fulfillment process that we could influence. Would you let me know when you are available this week?

Thanks,
Ayonija

In the above draft;

Notice the subject line ? Again, it's not precise. Then the writer doesn't get to the point of the communication until the last line. If the reader is scanning for information, he might not even get to the last line before moving on to the next email. If that happens, you'll have to write another communication or follow-up with a phone call - which is a waste of four time.

Now the good one:

Subject: Request to Meet with you regarding Sales Process-Please Respond.

Dear Vedant,

I'd like to meet you, the sales team and the marketing team this week want to discuss the impact of the latest sales trends on the launch of AquaRain Super. Would you be available on Monday at 3 pm for about an hour?

I spent some time with Divyanshi this morning reviewing the numbers from last quarter's sales results. I was concerned to see that there seems to be a downward trend in sales of the AquaRain, which is significantly different from what we forecasted. I think we should attempt to identify ant possible issues with the sales and fulfillment process.

Thanks,
Ayonija

See the difference ? The second email has a clear subject line that asks for a response. It gets to the point in the first paragraph. Even if the reader is scanning the information, he will have a better chance of getting the message.

Know your audience: When you are writing a communication, you need to be able to identify to whom you are writing. Sure, you could be writing to the 'world' of your organization or the 'world' of all of your customers, but you need to know what is that they will gain from your communication. Is it just information for everyone or are there particular unidentified members of the audience who need to receive your communication, recognize the information that is important to them, and then take a specific action.

For example, say you are changing the Life Insurance healthcare plan at the office so that domestic partners are now eligible for coverage. You might be sending the communication to everyone in your organization, but your true audience is employees that have domestic partners. In thinking about those people, what information do they need? What choices do they need to make? What concerns might they have in acting on the information? How can you handle those concerns in your communication? Identifying your audience helps you target and fine tune the communication in order to make it as effective as possible.

Another aspect of knowing your audience is being aware of what they don't know. Most of us have a 'lingo' that we use in the day to day operations of our work. They might be technical terms, references to internal structures or teams, or acronyms that are shared among peers. However, you need to be certain that every member of your audience would understand that lingo or acronym before using it, and that every person they might forward your communication to him so that they would understand it. When in doubt, add a brief explanation or spell it out.

Organization of the message: Perhaps your communication has more than one request or call to action. If the actions are unrelated to each other, the best choice is to send a separate email for each one. That requires your reader to see each topic in the subject line and then to respond accordingly.

However, you might have situations where you have several requests or several important facts for the reader. In that case, you need to organize the information in a way that increases the chance that the reader will give you all of the information or take all of the actions that you request. You can do this by using topic headings that still put the main topic of the communication at the top such as: Response Needed, Background, Concerns or RSVP Requested, Instructions, Directions, FAQs. You could also use bullets or numbers for each subtopic or consider using bold or coloured font to highlight requested actions. One word of caution-avoid using all capital letters, which can be interpreted as 'yelling'.

Your job is to make it easy and full-proof for your reader to get your message. Use whatever tools you can employ to ensure that the message is delivered fully, as long as still professional and appropriate for your audience.

EXERCISE

1.   'Writing skill is considered as one of the important communication skills'. Describe it.
2.   What is writing skill and why you think that this is a productive one.
3.   What is effective written communication ?
4.   What are the points one must keep in mind in order to write effectively?
5.   When and when not to use written communication, discuss with examples?

Chapter ... *8*

INTERVIEW SKILLS

♦ LEARNING OBJECTIVES ♦

Objectives of this chapter are:

- *to make the students able to understand the topic completely,*
- *to know do's and don'ts of interview skills,*
- *to appear in any interview confidently.*

8.1 PURPOSE OF AN INTERVIEW

Generally candidates are afraid of interviews as they think it to be a live ghost came to be faced. Remember that interview is nothing but a conversation, dialogue between two individuals who are at equal stature. In other words it is a method of getting an internal view of a candidate. So never think you are begging for a position, you are applying for it. Always feel relaxed while facing an interview as you need a job in the same way companies also need you. Always remember, first deserve then desire. Main purpose of the interview should be to attract and hire the best people available, not just hire the best people who apply. Before jumping ship to a new company, you inevitably need to test the waters during the job interview. The purpose of a job interview is twofold: It offers the employer valuable insight into your personality and abilities, and it allows you the chance to discern whether your credentials and career goals match up with what the company seeks. Job interviews can be quick -- sometimes lasting as little as a half hour -- or long, if you meet separately with two or more people from the company. When both parties listen intently and speak accurately, there is much to gain from the job-interview process.

Lets analyze candidates and employer's purposes separately.

The Employer's Purpose: Employers need to know three things about you:

- Can you do the work? Do you possess the skills and qualifications as reflected in your experience and education.
- Will you do the work? They need to know, based upon your interests and goals at this stage of your career, if you are motivated.

> - Will you fit in? They want to determine if you are a good fit with co-workers and if your values are in line with the company's culture and mission. All other factors being equal, many hiring managers base their decisions on likeability and fit.
>
>   **The Candidate's Purpose:** As a candidate, you need to:
>
> - Describe your skills and abilities to show that you can do the work.
>
> - Describe your interests and goals at this stage of your career to demonstrate that you are motivated and will do the work.
>
> - Learn as much as possible about the position and employer to determine if the job and the company's culture are a good fit with your skills, values, interests, and goals.

The four big purposes of a professional employment interview are: Accurately assess competency, fit and motivation; prevent good candidates from being improperly assessed. If you're a recruiter you've experienced this problem first hand many times. It happens whenever a fully-vetted candidate you've worked hard to find gets blown out because the hiring manager conducted a superficial or flawed assessment. If you've ever been on the interviewing team, you've experienced the problem second hand. This happens whenever there is wide disagreement about candidate competency among the members of the interviewing team. It means most of the interviewers are using either emotion, intuition, or some narrow range of factors to determine competency, fit and motivation to do the work. One countermeasure for this type of incorrect assessment is specific evidence disproving the false conclusion. For example, assuming that a soft-spoken person lacks team skills can be disproved by describing the big, multi-functional teams the person has been assigned to and asked to lead. Third purpose of interview is to clarify real job needs, demonstrate to the candidate that the assessment is professional, and that the company has extremely high hiring standards. Candidates – especially those with multiple opportunities – react negatively to box-checking, overt selling, superficial assessments and interviewers who are clueless when asked, "What's the focus of the job, and what are some of the challenges the person hired will face right away?" Conducting an in-depth performance-based interview using the Most Significant Accomplishment question eliminates these concerns. This structured approach not only clarifies real job expectations (the #1 driver of performance and job satisfaction), but also ensures the candidate fully appreciates the importance of the job, that he or she was properly evaluated, and that the company has high hiring standards. Fourth purpose is to shift the decision to career growth rather than compensation maximization. If this "career gap" (e.g., bigger team, bigger budget, better projects, more impact and exposure, faster growth, etc.) is big enough, compensation becomes less important. If the gap is too wide the candidate is too light for the job, and if the gap is too small, or non-existent, the job isn't big enough.

8.2 STEPS BEFORE GOING TO AN INTERVIEW

- Read the advertisement/ profile carefully.
- Visit the company's profile/website.
- Collect the news/ items related to the company.
- For you first few interviews, your background is important. Your school, medium, place (they give the interviewer an idea about you).
- Carry a copy of Resume/ Curriculum Vitae you have already sent and the interview letter. Keep an extra copy with you, just in case. Show interviewer letter to the receptionist / interviewer to establish your credentials. But keep this letter with you only for reference. The official addresses of the company for future correspondence are given on it.
- Carry everything you need for the interview in a neat folder. (never have loose papers cascading to the floor)
- Never carry your papers in a plastic/ cloth/shopping bag. Invest on a good folder, plastic or even leather.
- Never get your hair cropped just a day before interview or the same day. They may look awkward. If possible get them trimmed before 4-7 days so that by the day of interview they may come in a good shape.
- Don't feel shy or hesitant about calling up the and getting details about location, landmark, bus routes other information to help you reach the venue.
- If you are in the same town, go and 'ease the point' see where the venue is and how long will it take you to get there.
- Always arrive at least 15 minutes earlier before your time. It gives you time to catch your breath in case you climbed the stair too fast.
- Try to know if possible to know about the industry and its history in which it operates.
- Know about the current and international trends in the industry.
- Know about the mission/goals/philosophy/objective/motto/lobo etc. of the company.
- If possible know about the founder, member and CEO (Chief Executive Officer) and top management.
- Be careful about spellings and pronunciation.
- Know about the products and services of the company.
- Make a comparative study of the company and its competitors.
- Know the company's achievements, standards and certifications etc.
- Know about the hierarchy (system, group, branches, methods of writing).

- Know about the expectations from the offered job.
- Know about the remuneration standards for the job.
- Use gimmicks (Change your C.V./Resume) according to the company.
- Prepare thoroughly for the interview. If necessary mug some/ few answers (But give the answer with appropriate pause and modulations to give)
- Have some practice sessions with some close persons of yours.
- Talk to your people who have had experience of giving interviews for the similar position/post.
- Talk to the people who are working on the similar profile.
- Stick to the point.
- Be prepared for some irrelevant questions.

8.3 DO'S AND DON'TS FOR INTERVIEW

Attire (Dressing)

Dressing sense is the index of one's personality. What type of attire does a person like to wear depends largely upon his own personality. In interviews also the dressing sense matters a lot. So your dress and grooming send out powerful message to a prospective employer. The dressing as we notice is different in boys and girls. Here are some tips...

Attire for Men

- A conservative business suit is the best choice.
- Never wear black suit (it gives an impression as if you were in any funeral).
- Your clothes should be well stitched and appropriate for the occasion.
- If you appear clean, neat and polished, you make a good impression.
- Solid or pinstriped grey or navy blue, light cream light green shirt with grey shirt or white shirt is always a good investment.
- You can wear a navy blue shirt with grey trousers and shirt and black shoes and black belt.
- You can wear light green/cream shirt with greyer black trousers +black shoes+ black belt.
- If you are a fresh graduate and have you institute's blazer, it is a good combination with white shirt and grey trousers.
- Remember to wear a cotton vest or undershirt with your shirt even in hot weather, since it makes the shirt look brighter.
- As for the tie, it should be of silk, stripped or have small pattern as dots. Avoid large elaborate patterns or ties with too many colours.
- Avoid rings / bracelets and other ornaments as possible unless they are very personal to you.

Attire for Women

- Women will probably dress in a sari. Salwar kameez or a business suit. On no account should you wear jeans to the interviews.
- Choose silks in colder weather and cotton in summer.
- Classic patterns in navy blue grey or some dark, colour is in generally the best.
- Lighter pastoral shades are more common in summer.
- For certain jobs, especially for younger candidates dress may be preferred to a sari.
- You are never supported to go for an interview in a short skirt unless you are looking for a position in a fashion industry.
- In traditionally mate dominated fields such as banking and law, miniskirts and skirts with high slits are not advisable.
- Clinging clothes purple or glittery finger nails. Open toe shoes and dangling ear-rings are not preferred. But a pearl stud earrings and strand or pearl can add a touch of sophistication.
- The important thing is to wear just a few pieces of jewelry. Add one gold chain and a watch to your pearl set.
- Your nail polish should be clipped and clear in colour. Pink or red.
- Never wear red to an interview at financial institution or a conservative company.
- Carrying a small briefcase is optional but do not carry a causal shoulder bag or shopping bag.
- Sandals with saris and pumps with dress. If possible, select foot wear that conceal toes.
- Lady hats are not seen in India. Avoid them.
- Scent should be light and sweet just to avoid your body-odor don't use stinks.

What to Carry

Your interview invitation should detail everything that you need, but generally you should take:

- A bottle of water;
- An a-z street map, or at least the postcode of the organisation so that you can search google maps on your mobile phone;
- Details of the person that you must ask for upon arrival;
- Exam certificates, examples of your work, and any further evidence of your past successes; Money; Pen and notepad; Photo id (e.g. Passport or driving license);
- The job description and person specification;
- Your CV, letter of application and interview invitation;
- Your mobile phone but it switched off during the interview.

Steps During Interviews

The interview room appears to be a ghost for most of the candidates. But by following and practicing some simple tips, one can bring success to himself.

- Who you are, what you are interested in doing. Focus the job requirements and your accomplishments highlighting whoever the two matches.
- Instead of telling your qualities cite actual examples. (Your concrete achievements). Keep these memories handy so that you can recount them at the proper time.
- You should actually seek opportunities to insert these self-advertisements during the interview.
- Mirror the style and pace of your interviewer. The he is friendly and chatty try to be the same. On the other hand if he/she is formal and uses quick fire questions, respond in the same way.
- Show interest in company, the job, especially the employer.
- Mind you are not fully dressed unless you put on a smile.
- Don't anticipate questions and don't interrupt the interviewer.
- Present a profile of yourself in less than two minutes. It is like a two minutes commercial.
- Convey enthusiasm and warmth, but not the back slapping. Kind of friendship.
- Maintain eye contact but don't try to stare the interviewer.
- Prove yourself capable of performing rather than merely describing. Provide concrete examples that illustrate the success you have achieved so far.
- Use natural gestures and avoid fidgeting.
- Ensure that you speak clearly and with well molded voice that supports appropriate excitement for the opportunity before you.
- You should relaxed and confident. After all just as you need a job, the employer also needs a good employer polite, positive and passionate.
- Don't fabricate, guess or generalise and don't get involved in a debate with the interviewer.
- Follow up with an effective 'Thank You' letter. Don't write this letter lightly. It is another opportunity to market yourself.
- Find some areas discussed in the meeting and expand them in the letter after the meeting, is minimum. So consider this letter as an additional interview.

Body Language During Interview:

Do's

- **Walk in confidently:** As soon as you walk into the building you'll begin to be judged on your behaviour.

- **Deliver a firm handshake:** Come on too weak and you'll seem submissive, but come on too strong and you could be seen to be trying too hard. Keep it firm, but try not to crush their fingers.

- **Sit up straight:** Avoid being too stiff, but try to sit up straight, keeping the small of your back against the chair.

- **Maintain eye contact:** Maintaining eye contact shows the interviewer you're not intimidated, and that you're taking everything in. If you feel uncomfortable, look away for a few seconds or try looking at their nose.

- **Smile:** Recruiters seldom employ miserable people. It's ok to be nervous, but a smile can go a long way. It makes you look more relaxed, comfortable and personable. To put it simply, it will make you more likeable

- **Watch your hands:** Keep your arms uncrossed and your hands away from your face (touching your nose or ear is sometimes said to indicate lying

Don'ts

- **Be overconfident:** Arrogance is not a good look. Remember: arrogance and confidence is not the same thing.

- **Offer a weak handshake:** Try and mirror your interviewer's handshake, and apply the same amount of pressure.

- **Slouch:** Bad posture can make you look bored and uninterested. Effectively, you are closing yourself off from the situation.

- **Stare:** It's always important to maintain eye contact, but there's definitely a limit. Don't make it too intense.

- **Play with Your Pen/Hair:** Really think about this one. It seems so obvious, but as with most body language, you often don't know you're doing it. Be aware of any bad habits you have before your interview, and keep them in the back of your mind.

- **Fidget :** Try to avoid moving around too much. Nervously moving your feet or constantly changing position will only make you look awkward and uncomfortable.

Tips For Controlling Your Nerves

It is but natural that a candidate going to face an interview is a little bit nervous. But nervousness may cause a hurdle in his success and selection. Nerves can make you forget to do things as simple as listening. This can result in you being thought of as unfriendly or inattentive. So here are some tips to overcome nervousness. Though it is not possible to master this in one day, a regular practice before some days from the interview will help a lot. Here are some ideas for combating nerves include:

- Being aware of the interview's structure, and the fact that they often begin with easier questions such as 'tell us about your time at university';
- Exercising before your interview, as this burns off negative energy and creates feelings of wellbeing;
- Pausing before answering a difficult question to give yourself thinking time, or asking for clarification if, at first, you're unsure what the question means;
- Putting everything into perspective, reminding yourself that the worst thing that can happen is you not getting the job;
  - ➢ Taking a toilet break before the interview;
  - ➢ Taking deep breaths and not speaking too quickly;
  - ➢ Taking notes with you, writing down cues to highlight examples that you want to draw upon;
  - ➢ Thinking about positive and happy experiences before the interview starts, and visualising yourself in complete control during the interview.

Some Common Questions Asked During Interviews:

- Tell us about yourself.
- What are your short term and long term goals? / What are your goals?
- What are your future aspects?
- What do you like doing most?
- Do you prefer to work by yourself or with others?
- What are your hobbies?
- What are your strengths and weaknesses?
- How do you learn of our company?
- What do you know want to work for the company?
- Tell me about your previous job experience.
- Why did you leave your previous job experience? / Tell about your previous job.
- Why should we hire you?
- Why do you want to work here?
- Why are you looking for another position?
- Why did you leave your previous position?
- What are your best skills?
- What have been your major achievements?
- What type of management style do you work best with?

- What would your current manager/ boss say about you?

- In your most recent position, what have been your most significant achievements?

- What motivates you in the work environment?

- What frustrates you in the work environment?

- How would you describe your own personality?

- What areas have you identified that you would like to improve and what have you done about them?

- What are your career goals?

- What levels of salary are you seeking? / What salary are you expecting?

8.4 TELEPHONIC INTERVIEWS

These are usually used for cost-efficient preliminary screening before the first one-to-one interview. They're often recorded and vary in length, but average around 20-30 minutes. You should prepare for a phone interview just as you would for a regular interview and generally should:

- Direct the interviewer to your web portfolio or link in profile if possible, to demonstrate your work in practice;

- Find a quiet place for the interview where you'll be undisturbed;

- Fully charge your mobile before the interview, and turn call waiting off;

- Get your main messages across quickly, by writing down your key attributes and having these at hand during the call;

- Have a glass of water available;

- Have a pen and notepad within reach;

- Have internet access;

- Keep your CV, application and job description in clear view;

- Not interrupt the interviewer;

- Not smoke, chew gum or eat;

- Smile, as this projects a positive image and changes your tone of voice;

- Speak slowly and clearly;

- Take time to collect your thoughts, and give relatively short answers.

Video interviews are increasingly common, especially if you're applying for overseas jobs. Remember to dress as you would for a face-to-face interview, and check your background before the interview begins. Finally, ensure that your body language is positive; look directly into the camera and make eye contact, as this'll make you appear calm and confident.

EXERCISE

1. What is an interview?

2. What is the purpose of conducting an interview?

3. What are common points to be kept in mind while appearing in an interview?

4. "Body language plays very crucial role during interview", discuss this with valid examples.

5. What may be appropriate answer of the question 'Describe yourself', asked during an interview?

6. How to answer different questions asked during an interview?

Chapter ... 9

GIVING PRESENTATIONS

♦ LEARNING OBJECTIVES ♦

Objectives of this chapter are:

- *To make the students able to understand basic concept of presentation.*
- *To learn about effective body language which is to be maintained during presentation.*
- *To deliver presentation nicely and effectively in front of different types of audiences.*

9.1 INTRODUCTION

Presentation is the process of presenting the content of a topic to the audience when the presentation is made by oral means, it can be termed as oral presentation. An oral presentation is formal, structured and systematic presentation of a message / topic to the audience. It involves conveying lot of information in a limited time. There are two main types of oral presentation; Extempore and Prepared oral presentation.

Extempore: In extempore topic is given at the last moment and time duration is also very short.

Prepared Oral Presentation: In prepared oral presentation you know the topic, your audience and the time limit beforehand. So that you can prepare and get relevant reference material to prepare the final draft of you presentation. Even you can edit it properly.

Oral presentation is a form of oral communication. It is a participative two-way communicative process characterized by the formal and structured presentation of a message using visual aids. Making a good oral presentation is an art that involves attention to the needs of your audience, careful planning, and attention to delivery. It also covers use of notes, visual aids and computer presentation software.

Importance of Oral Presentation: Oral presentation plays a vital role in modern business. Successful oral presentation can boost the career of an employee while failure to present well, can hinder the career growth. Oral presentation is important for the following reasons:

- A professional student may be required to make presentation in the form of progress report, students' seminars, research presentations etc.
- Professionals like scientists and Engineers has to make oral reports, present seminars, delivers presentations on research projects and etc.
- A business executive has to make presentation to introduce a news product that their company has launched.
- Oral presentation is a tool of professional and business interaction.
- This skill contributes to professional success.
- Oral presentation is the basis of selection process.
- It may help in getting lucrative job.
- It may help to get a big business deal.
- To get the promotion.
- Oral presentation is helpful in group discussion, interviews and paper presentation.

9.2 DEALING WITH FEARS

Stage fright is the fear of crowd or stage. Symptoms of stage fright are stammering, sweating, shivering, increased rate of heart beat ,drying of mouth ,forgetting the entire matter etc. We can overcome our stage fright just by following few points given below;

- Set realistic goals.
- Avoid negative thoughts.
- Speak slowly and confidently.
- Concentrate on three P's i.e. planning, preparation and practice .
- Fully prepare the final draft of the presentation.
- Start with confidence.
- Pay attention to body language and try to maintain eye contact.
- Learn and practice stress reduction techniques.
- To gain confidence watch successful presentations of other speakers.

9.3 PLANNING YOUR PRESENTATION

There are four P's related with oral presentation. These are Planning, Preparation, Practice and Performance or Presentation.

- **Planning:** Here we define the purpose, analyze the audience and occasion and choose appropriate title of the presentation.
- **Preparation:** Here relevant material is collected from reliable sources and resources available. Later on it is organized properly either chronologically or logically, now rough draft is ready. After reading and re-reading rough draft is edited and final draft is prepared.

- **Practice:** Rehearsing the prepared presentation again and again.
- **Performance:** Final delivery of presentation.

In an effective presentation, the content and structure are adjusted to the medium of speech. When listening, we cannot go back over a difficult point to understand it or easily absorb long arguments. A presentation can easily be ruined if the content is too difficult for the audience to follow or if the structure is too complicated. As a general rule, expect to cover much less content than you would in a written report. Make difficult points easier to understand by preparing the listener for them, using plenty of examples and going back over them later. Leave time for questions within the presentation. Give your presentation a simple and logical structure. Include an introduction in which you outline the points you intend to cover and a conclusion in which you go over the main points of your talk.

The audience: Some basic questions to ask about an audience are:

1. Who will I be speaking to?
2. What do they know about my topic already?
3. What will they want to know about my topic?
4. What do I want them to know by the end of my talk?

By basing the content and style of your presentation on your answers to these questions, you can make sure that you are in tune with your audience. What you want to say about your topic may be much less important than what your audience wants to hear about it.

Content: It is likely that you already have a topic and you know what you want to say about it. This is the content of your presentation. You may already have the content of your presentation in written form: for example in a written report. Whether your content is already written down or you are beginning from scratch, you may need to cut it down for your presentation. Why?

- You will need to fit your content within the time limit. Think carefully about how much information you can reasonably present in the time allowed and select the most important point.
- You will need to hold the interest and attention of your audience. Many people lose interest towards the end of presentations that contain too much information. Think carefully about the key points that you want to get across and build your presentation around them.
- Some kinds of information, such as technical explanations and tables of figures, are difficult for listeners to absorb during a presentation. Think about summarising this kind of information or referring the listeners to a document they can read after the presentation.
- You will need to leave time for examples and illustrations of your points. Think carefully about how you will support and explain your key points.

- You will need to leave time for an introduction, conclusion and questions or comments. During this time you are likely to be repeating points made in the main body of your talk.

Three points to think about when preparing the content of a presentation:

- What are your key points? Most good presentations have no more than 5 key points.
- How will you support your key points with examples and illustrations?
- How will you make it easy for your audience to follow your key points?

9.4 STRUCTURING YOUR PRESENTATION

Most presentations will consist of an introduction, the body of the talk and a conclusion. The introduction prepares the audience for what you will say in the body of the talk and the conclusion reminds them of your key points. Good presentations raise questions in the listeners' mind. Good speakers encourage questions both during and after the presentation and are prepared to answer them.

Introduction: A good introduction does four things:

- Attracts and focuses the attention of the audience.
- Puts the speaker and audience at ease.
- Explains the purpose of the talk and what the speaker would like to achieve.
- Gives an overview of the key points of the talk.

It is often a good idea to begin a talk with a question, a short story, an interesting fact about your topic or an unusual visual aid. Many speakers follow this with an overhead transparency that shows the title, aim and outline of the talk.

Body: The body of a presentation must be presented in a logical order that is easy for the audience to follow and natural to your topic. Divide your content into sections and make sure that the audience knows where they are at any time during your talk. It is often a good idea to pause between main sections of your talk. You can ask for questions, sum up the point or explain what the next point will be. If you have an OHT with an outline of your talk on it, you can put this on the projector briefly and point to the next section.

Examples, details and visual aids add interest to a presentation and help you get your message through. Here are some questions you can ask yourself about the examples you include:

- Are they relevant to the experience of the audience?
- Are they concrete?
- Will the audience find them interesting?
- Are they varied?
- Are they memorable?

Conclusion: A good conclusion does two things:

- Reminds the audience of your key points.
- Reinforces your message

Your conclusion should end the presentation on a positive note and make the audience feel that have used their time well listening to you.

Questions: Many speakers worry about questions from the audience. However, questions show that the audience is interested in what you have to say ad can make the talk more lively and interactive. You should be more worried if there are no questions at all! One way of handling questions is to point to questions you would like to discuss as you are talking. You can control questions better if you leave pauses during your talk and ask for questions. It is important not to let question and answer sessions during the talk go on too long, however. Answer briefly or say you will deal with the question at the end. Make sure you are ready to go on with your talk when questions have finished.

Visual aids: Visual aids help to make a presentation more lively. They can also help the audience to follow your presentation and help you to present information that would be difficult to follow through speech alone. The two most common forms of visual aid are overhead transparencies (OHTs) and computer slide shows (e.g. PowerPoint). Objects that can be displayed or passed round the audience can also be very effective and often help to relax the audience. Some speakers give printed handouts to the audience to follow as they speak. Others prefer to give their handouts at the end of the talk, because they can distract the audience from the presentation. Visual aids can be a very powerful tool to enhance the impact of your presentations. Words and images presented in different formats can appeal directly to your audience's imagination, adding power to your spoken words.

Think of using visual aids for the following reasons:

- If they will save words - don't describe your results - show them;
- If their impact would be greater than the spoken word - don't describe an image - show it.

Think about using a variety of different visual images. Try using photographs, tables, diagrams, charts, drawings, key words, or video sequences. Be creative and deliberate in your choice of images to achieve the most impact. Think of your next presentation. How can you display your material visually? What techniques might help you present your argument or results in a stimulating way? What might add emphasis to your spoken words?

Use of Audio Visual Aids: A presentation of statistical data, figures and diagrams and so on is made vivid by the use of visual aids. Though visual display of ideas, we make our audience see what they hear. We help the listeners receive our message effortlessly. Visual aids should be used to:

- Present data which is numerical or statistical.
- Display of material like art, design or any subject.

- Present comparative statements of facts and figures, especially graphic and diagrammatic forms.
- Present a new plan or new concept which will be more effective through visual aids.
- Comparative studies of past and present data.

Advantages of Using Audio Visual Aids in Oral Presentation: Use of audio visual aids in oral presentation is having following advantages;

- Information communicated through visual aids is retained for a very long time, because when a person sees and hears a thing at the same time, the impact is much greater.
- The combination of visual image and the message is an attention getter. It develops interest and attracts the attention of the audience.
- When he makes use of effectiveness of the presenter is also increased due to visual aids. The presenter feels more confident and sure of himself when he makes use of visual aids.

When to Use Visual Aids: Words and images can be used throughout your presentation from the introduction to the conclusion. However, remember to restrict their use to key moments in your presentation; an over use of visual aids can be hard to follow.

Think about using visual aids at the following times:

Time of using Visual Aids	**Ways of Using Visual Aids**
Introduction	<ul><li>Display the title of your presentation;</li><li>Define particular technical terms or units;</li><li>Indicate a structure to your presentation by listing your main points;</li><li>Display an image which encapsulates your theme(s);</li><li>Highlight a question you intend answering during the course of your presentation;</li></ul>
Main Points	<ul><li>Highlight new points with an appropriate image or phrase;</li><li>Support technical information with clearly displayed data;</li><li>Indicate sequence by linking points together;</li><li>Offer evidence from your research to support your argument;</li></ul>

Time of using Visual Aids	Ways of Using Visual Aids
Conclusion	<ul><li>Summaries your main points on a slide;</li><li>Present your conclusion in a succinct phrase or image;</li><li>Display your key references to allow your audience to read more on your topic.</li></ul>

Designing visual aids: There are many different rules for designing visual aids, some of which will apply directly to different kinds of equipment. In general, sticking to the following guidelines will produce high quality visual images:

- Use one simple idea for each visual;
- Make the text and diagrams clear and readable;
- Avoid cluttering the image;
- Keep your images consistent (use the same font, titles, lay out etc. for each image);
- Make sure your images are of a high quality (check for spelling and other errors).
- Use visual aids (text, graphs, charts, tables, illustrations, etc.) to clarify your presentation, not as a basis for it.
- Keep visual aids uncluttered. Research shows that people cannot listen to a presentation and process visual aids that are too heavy with text or data.
- Use bulleted text.
- Use simple layout/design.
- Keep graphs, charts, and tables easy to "read" and interpret
- Use titles on each visual aid to guide the audience.
- Make sure that the font size is legible from all seats.
- Have paper copies of slides or transparencies to distribute in the event of a technical difficulty.
- Make sure that every slide or transparency can stand on its own (i.e., out of context with the other slides/transparencies and the presentation itself).

Do and Don't of Oral Presentation

- Use a big enough font (minimum 20 pt).
- Make it so small you can't read it.
- Keep the background simple.
- Use a fussy background image.
- Use animations when appropriate.
- Don't over-do the animation - it gets distracting.

- Make things visual.
- Use endless slides of bulleted lists that all look the same.
- For more detailed guidance see the Using PowerPoint study guide.

9.5 DELIVERING YOUR PRESENTATION

People vary in their ability to speak confidently in public, but everyone gets nervous and everyone can learn how to improve their presentation skills by applying a few simple techniques. The main points to pay attention to in delivery are the quality of your voice, your rapport with the audience, use of notes and use of visual aids. Voice quality involves attention to volume, speed and fluency, clarity and pronunciation. The quality of your voice in a presentation will improve dramatically if you are able to practice beforehand in a room similar to the one you will be presenting in. Rapport with the audience involves attention to eye contact, sensitivity to how the audience is responding to your talk and what you look like from the point of view of the audience. These can be improved by practicing in front of one or two friends or video-taping your rehearsal.

Voice Quality: Your voice is your main channel of communication to the audience, so make sure you use it to its best effect.

Volume: Is your voice loud enough or too loud? Adjust your volume to the size of the room and make sure the people at the back can hear. In a big room take deep breaths and try to project your voice rather than shout.

Speed and Fluency: Speak at a rate so your audience can understand your points. Do not speed up because you have too much material to fit into the time available. Try not to leave long pauses while you are looking at your notes or use fillers such as 'um' or 'er'. Use pauses to allow the audience to digest an important point. Repeat or rephrase difficult or important points to make sure the audience understands.

Clarity: Speak clearly. Face the audience and hold your head up. Your speech will be clearer if you look directly at the members of the audience while you speak. Keep your hands and notes away from your mouth and keep your eyes on the audience when you are talking about overhead transparencies. If you have to look at the whiteboard or the overhead projector, stop talking until you are ready to face the audience again.

Pronunciation: You may not be able to improve your general pronunciation much before an important presentation. However, you can make sure you know how to pronounce names and difficult words. Do not use exaggerated intonation or pronunciation of individual words. Your natural speaking style will be good enough as long as you speak clearly.

Engaging the Audience: One of the secrets of a good presentation is to involve the audience.

Maintain Eye Contact: Look your audience in the eyes. Spread your eye contact around the audience including those at the back and sides of the room. Avoid looking at anyone too long because this can be intimidating!

Ask for Feedback: You can involve the audience by asking occasional questions. Try to ask genuine questions to which you do not already know the answer and show interest in any replies. Leave time for the audience to think and try to avoid answering your questions yourself or telling members of the audience that their answers are wrong. Questions to the audience work well when you manage to make those who answer them feel that they have contributed to your presentation.

You can also pause occasionally to ask if anyone has any questions for you. If a question disrupts the flow of your talk too much, you can say that you will answer it later (but don't forget to do it!). Before you ask for questions, make sure you are ready to pick up your presentation again when the Q & A session has finished.

Look Confident: It is natural to feel nervous in front of an audience. Experienced speakers avoid looking nervous by breathing deeply, speaking slowly and avoiding unnecessary gestures or movements. Smiling and focusing attention on members of the audience who show interest can also help you feel more confident as your talk progresses.

Effective Use of Notes: Good speakers vary a great deal in their use of notes. Some do not use notes at all and some write out their talk in great detail. If you are not an experienced speaker it is not a good idea to speak without notes because you will soon lose your thread. You should also avoid reading a prepared text aloud or memorizing your speech as this will be boring. The best solution may be to use notes with headings and points to be covered. You may also want to write down key sentences. Notes can be on paper or cards. Some speakers use overhead transparencies as notes. The trick in using notes is to avoid shifting your attention from the audience for too long. Your notes should always be written large enough for you to see without moving your head too much. One of the decisions you have to make before you give a presentation is how to remember what you are going to say. Experienced presenters use a variety of methods. On this page we outline the advantages and disadvantages of each. It is up to you to decide which is best for you.

Speaking Without Notes: Some presenters do not use notes at all. They just remember the outline of what they are going to say and talk.

Advantages: If you do it well, you will seem natural, knowledgeable and confident of your topic. You will also find it easier to establish rapport with the audience because you can give them your full attention.

Disadvantages: It is easy to lose your thread, miss out whole sections of your talk or to go over the time limit. People who speak without notes often fail to convey a clear idea of the structure of their ideas to the audience.

This is a high-risk strategy. A few people can present effectively without notes. If you are one of them, good luck!

Reading from a Script: Some experienced presenters write down every word they intend to say. They may read the whole script aloud or they may just use it as a back-up.

Advantages: You will find it easier to keep within the time limit. You are likely to less nervous and make fewer mistakes.

Disadvantages: It is difficult to establish rapport with the audience. You may sound like you are reading aloud rather than speaking to an audience. Listeners often lose interest in a presentation that is read aloud.

This is a low-risk strategy employed by many experienced non-native speaker presenters. If you use it, you will need to develop the skill of reading aloud while still sounding natural. Few people can do this effectively.

Note cards: Many presenters write down headings and key points on cards or paper. They use them as reminders of what they are going to say.

Advantages: You will find it easier to establish rapport with the audience. Your presentation will be structured but you will sound natural.

Disadvantages: You may find it difficult to keep within the time limit. If your notes are too brief, you may forget what you intended to say.

This is a medium-risk strategy used by many experienced presenters and the one most often recommended. The disadvantages of note cards can be overcome if you practice your presentation before you give it.

Overhead Transparencies: Some presenters use their OHTs as notes. They use them like note cards as reminders of what they are going to say. Handouts and PowerPoint presentations can be used in the same way.

Advantages: It is easy to establish rapport with the audience because you are sharing your notes with them. You will sound natural and your presentation will seem well-organised.

Disadvantages: You may find it difficult to keep within the time limit. Your presentation may be dominated by your OHTs. Unless you are careful, you may find that you are talking to the overhead projector rather than the audience.

This is a medium-to-high-risk strategy. Used well, it can be very effective, especially by presenters who are used to speaking without notes.

9.6 TECHNIQUES OF DELIVERY

Presentation means speaking before people on some formal occasion. It is an essential feature of one's professional life. The good delivering of presentation requires certain techniques, these are;

- Use of proper grammar.
- Use of proper syntax.
- Use of the simplest and appropriate words.
- Avoidance of imperfect words or jargons.
- Ability to pronounce words correctly.

- Use of clear voice.
- Use of proper pauses to either highlight the punctuation or to create effect.
- Proper use of intonation.
- Use of steady pace, which is neither too fast nor too slow.
- Be positive, firm and relaxed.
- Structure your presentation.
- Do not read from script.
- Use note-cards.
- Use appropriate visual aids.
- Do not go over the allotted time.
- Pay attention to body language-effective posture and gestures etc.
- Maintain eye contact.
- Close ion a memorable way.

Barriers to Effective Presentation:

Following points may act as a barrier to effective presentation;

- Lack of preparation of the topic.
- Reliance on one source only.
- Absence of self confidence.
- Mispronunciation of the new words.
- Absence of clarity of voice.
- Negligence of effective body movement.
- Presence of stage fright.
- Presence of negative thoughts.
- Lack of practice.

Ten Steps to Preparing an Effective Oral Presentation

- Determine the purpose of your presentation and identify your own objectives.
- Know your audience and what it knows.
- Define your topic.
- Arrange your material in a way that makes sense for your objectives.
- Compose your presentation.
- Create visual aids.
- Practice your presentation (don't forget to time it.
- Make necessary adjustments.
- Analyze the room where you'll be giving your presentation (set-up, sight lines, equipment, etc.)

EXERCISE

1.   What is the difference between extempore and oral presentation.

2.   What are four P's of oral presentation?

3.   What points makes your presentation effective?

4.   How AV aids are helpful in making your presentation impressive?

5.   What is stage freight and how could you overcome it?

6.   What points are to be considered while preparing your slides for presentation ?

Chapter ... **10**

GROUP DISCUSSION

♦ LEARNING OBJECTIVES ♦

Objectives of this chapter are:

- *to make the students able to understand basic concept of group discussion.*
- *to learn different types of group discussions.*
- *to understand different do's and don'ts of group discussion.*
- *to participate in group discussions, to present their views nicely in front of others.*

10.1 INTRODUCTION

Group Discussion is a systematic and purposeful interactive oral process that is widely used to evaluate several candidates simultaneously as a variant personality test. The other purpose of conducting group discussion is to test the presentation skills and public speaking skills of a candidate so that suitable candidates may be short listed for the final interview. The literal meaning of the word 'discuss' is *'to talk about a given subject in detail'*. So in other words it can be considered as a systematic oral exchange of information, views and opinions to other participants and thereby come to a consensus or conclusion.

Types of Group Discussion:

Group Discussions are of different types depending upon the subject and subject matter. Basically there are three types of group Discussions. Topic based GDs can be classified into four groups: The group discussions can be classified under two heads:

Topic Based Group discussions: In this type of group discussions, participants are asked to share their views on the given topic and finally they are evaluated on the basis of the views they put forth. These topics may be based on different issues like Current affairs, Factual topics, Controversial topics and Abstract topics.

Current Affairs or Factual Topics

Current Affair is the affair that has been in the news recently. These topics are given to judge analytical skills and general awareness of the candidate.

Factual Topics

Topics are related to socio-economic, practical day to day topics, politics of Indian education, culture etc. They are about practical things, which an ordinary person is aware of in his day-to-day life. A candidate is given a chance to prove that he is aware and has good knowledge. These topics may be based on socio-economic and general topics.

Controversial Topics

Controversial topics are the ones that are argumentative in nature. They are meant to check maturity and logic in a person. For example, *should reservations be there or not?"* In GDs where these topics are given for discussion, the noise level is usually high, there may be tempers flying. The idea behind giving a topic like this is to see how much maturity the candidate is displaying by keeping his temper in check, by rationally and logically arguing his point of view without getting personal and emotional.

Abstract Topics

Abstract topics are about intangible things. They are given to check creativity and lateral thinking. For example *Black shoes pink laces, Talk about number 13, misfortune is a fortune in disguise etc*. These topics are not given often for discussion, but their possibility cannot be ruled out.

Case based Group Discussion: In a Case Study GD, case-lets dealing with real life situation in the corporate world are given for discussion. In this type of group discussion, first the candidates are asked to read the case properly. They are given a set of information, a situation, a problem and they are expected to produce the probable solution of the case. After that, they are required to share their views on the basis of their evaluations analysis of the case and discuss on the basis of the points with the group members.

These types of Group discussions are very popular in many B- schools, IIMs etc. Here, the candidate is required to study the case and then discuss the same among the group. Such discussions try to simulate real-life situation which are generally problematic and there are no incorrect answers or perfect solutions. It enables the candidates to think from various angles.

10.2 COMMUNICATION SKILLS IN A GROUP DISCUSSION

To communicate means to interact. Communication skills means all those skills which helps us to express our views properly in front of others. Group discussion plays a significant role in the life of a student. It is a forum for discussing a topic with common objective of finding a solution for a problem or discussing on an issue. Nowadays, group discussion has attained very much importance as selection criterion for admission in business schools and professional organizations. There are many reasons behind the increasing importance of GDs in campus selections. Its contribution to the academics can be understood from the following points:

- It is a tool to test how effectively an individual is able to participate in a group or he contributes towards group objectives.

- It is also an effective tool to test how well does an individual listen to others' points of view.

- They are helpful to check how open minded a participant is towards accepting contrary views and criticism.

- The examiner checks how does a participant control his emotions in case of any wrong comment.

- It helps the student to train himself to discuss and argue about the topic given.

- It helps him to express his views on serious subjects and in formal situations.

- It improves his thinking, listening and speaking skills besides promoting his confidence level.

- It is an effective tool in problem solving, decision making and personality assessment.

- GD skills may ensure academic success, popularity and good admission or job offer.

- Most importantly it checks other important personality traits like confidence, self discipline, self motivation, leadership skills, cooperative nature etc of a participant

After going through the above mentioned points we can say that it is important to be able to take part in a GD effectively and confidently. Participants should know how to speak with confidence, how to exhibit leadership skills and how to make the group attain the common goals.

10.3 ESSENTIALS OF GROUP DISCUSSION

Clarity of Topic: When the topic of the group discussion is announced, one must move the vehicles of his/her own memory to gather all the points one can recollect. If one is totally unaware about the topic, one must not step ahead and initiate. He must first listen to the views of other, then understand the topic and then put forth his/her views.

Start where Left: Start the discussion from where the other person has left the topic. Do not just start giving your views. Try to synchronies your views with the views of other. Try to show agreement with others if you are satisfied with the points else you can put forth your views on disagreement.

Active Participation: One must actively participate in the group discussion to have a good impression on the jury as well as the fellow members. but this active participation should be emulsified with relevant views. Unnecessary and irrelevant points can put you in trouble and deduct the points. So be careful with your views.

Healthy Tone: Try to put forward your views in healthy and impressive tone. Do not get aggressive when anybody opposes you or is against your point. It also reduces the points. Remain calm and cool.

Keep eye contact while speaking: Do not look at the evaluators only. Keep eye contact with every team member while speaking.

Initiate the GD: Initiating the GD is a big plus. But keep in mind – Initiate the group discussion only when you understood the GD topic clearly and have some topic knowledge. Speaking without proper subject knowledge is bad impression.

Allow others to speak: Do not interrupt anyone in-between while speaking. Even if you don't agree with his/her thoughts do not snatch their chance to speak. Instead make some notes and clear the points when it's your turn.

Speak clearly: Speak politely. Use simple and understandable words while speaking. Don't be too aggressive if you are disagreeing with someone. Express your feelings calmly and politely.

Make sure to bring the discussion on track: it is essential to stick to your topic. So if by any means group is distracting from the topic or goal, then take initiative to bring the discussion on the track. Make all the members so that some conclusion is made at the end of the discussion.

Positive Attitude: Be confident. It is a negative trait to try to dominate anyone in the discussion. Keep positive language. Show interest in discussion. Be careful that your words don't hurt anyone's emotions.

Sensibly: Don't speak just to increase your speaking time. Don't worry even if you speak less. What matters is that your thoughts should be sensible and relevant to the topic.

Be a good listener: It is rightly said that only a good listener can be a good speaker. So listen carefully what other contestants say. This will make coherent discussion and you will get involved in the group positively. You will surely make people agree with you.

Be to the point: Some basic analysis is sufficient. No need to mention exact figures while giving any reference. As you have less time, it is better to be precise and convey your thoughts in short and simple language possible.

Dressing: Be careful that you should not be fancy and funny in your dressing. Dress yourself in a comfortable while speaking in group. Positive gestures and body language will make your work easy.

How to prepare for Group Discussion:

- If you are given a role which you are supposed to play at the end of the case, let them in such a scenario. You should look at the problem from its angle, and then discuss the case accordingly.

- In case you are to discuss it from a third party point of view, then look at it in a more holistic way. In case, the case is not specific in this regard, then you could assume the role of a third-party, look at the case objectively from all angles, and discuss it likewise.

- Try to include SWOT Analysis - Strengths, Weaknesses, Opportunities and Threats; while discussing the case study because you will need to develop and present a framework.

- Identify the main problem in the case and its possible causes. At first you will have to understand what the problem is and exactly which the area you need to look at is.

- Now on the basis of the problem, come up with two to three possible logical and analytical solutions that you think will work for the particular situation.

- Analyse the pros and cons of the solutions or suggestions you have made. Then choose the most feasible option to approach.

Difference between a Group Discussion and a Debate:

Most of the people take Group discussion and Debates as two names of same thing, but they are entirely different from each other. Of course it is an issue that is discussed in both type of mutual exchange of talks and opinions but they are different in many issues.

A debate is a form of discussion where there are usually two speakers exchanging their views on a subject or several public issues. Speakers speak as they counter the points raised by others with the help of their arguments. An audience is a part of the debate in the form of listeners, and there is no input from the audiences. Debates are meant to be constructive through an exchange of ideas but usually it is seen that speakers try to score brownie points over each other as also to win over audiences making it a destructive debate. However, the basic purpose of a debate is healthy exchange of ideas and opinions.

In schools and colleges, debating is an art of public speaking where the contestants are encouraged to exchange their ideas and opinions freely, taking turns to speak and counter the points raised by other contestants.

Base	Debate	Group Discussion
NATURE	Debate is competitive in nature and so is argumentative.	While group discussion is a co-operative group process and communication of ideals.
	Debates are destructive as they present one-sided opinions and demolish reasoned arguments,	Whereas discussions are constructive and encourage the expression of opinion.
SIDE	In a debate, a speaker can speak either 'for' the topic or 'against' the topic	Whereas in a GD, the speaker can express both.
DECISION	The final decision or result in a debate depends on voting	While in a GD, the group reaches group consensus
UNDERSTANDING	Debate is for argument and to attack to win	While group discussion is to exchange ideas and opinions for a better understanding of a topic.
TURNS/ SIDES	In a debate, speakers take turns to present their points	While, in a group discussion, all participants can discuss a topic presenting their opinions without turns.
DEFEND AN ATTACK	In a debate, a speaker has to defend or attack to win.	While, The views of all participants matter in a group discussion.

Some Positive and Negative Traits in Group Discussion:

POINTS THAT ARE CONSIDERED	POSITIVE TRAITS	NEGATIVE TRAITS
PERSONALITY TRAITS	Smartness, Cheerfulness, Enthusiasm, Keenness, Curiosity, appearance,	Shyness, sluggishness, nervousness, Difference, Timidity, Rudeness etc.

POINTS THAT ARE CONSIDERED	POSITIVE TRAITS	NEGATIVE TRAITS
	temperament. Gestures, mental status, participation etc.	
COMMUNICATION SKILLS	Listening skills, language, pronunciation, Fluency, Clarity of thoughts, Logical ability etc.	Muteness, Aggressiveness, Vagueness, Incoherence, Fumbling, Tonal Poverty (low volume).
KNOWLEDGE OF THE TOPIC	Depth, Range, Analytical Ability, Coordination of Thoughts.	Ignorance, Lack of Ideas, Superficiality, Incoherence, Lack of Analytical Ability
INTRA- INTERPERSONAL SKILLS/ LEADERSHIP SKILLS	Initiative, Tolerance, Team Spirit, Persuasiveness, Decisiveness, Flexibility, Friendliness.	Intolerance, Isolation. Unfriendliness, Rigidity, Selfishness.

Some Do's and Don'ts in Group Discussion:

Sr. No	Do's	Don'ts
1.	Seat yourself comfortably discussing	Be in a hurry to start
2.	Listen to the topic carefully	Be silent
3.	Organize your ideas before speaking	Dominate – vocally
4.	Speak at the earliest opportunity	Assume the role of the Chairman
5.	Be polite	Take extreme stance
6.	Identify your supporters and opponents	Enter into an argument.
7.	Allow your supporters to augment you're your ideas	Pass value judgment
8.	Keep track of time	Look at the faculty
9.	Share time fairly	Shout down inert participants
10.	Listen to others points	Move excessively in your chair or lean on the table.

Sr. No	Do's	Don'ts
11.		Dominating Nature
12.		Disagreeing beyond reasons
13.		Being relevant
14.		Losing temper
15.		Impatient Attitude
16.		Poor Communication Skills
17.		Ignorance about the topic given
18.		Non-Participation

Some Qualities Evaluated in Group Discussion:

There are some essential points that every participant of the discussion should necessarily keep in mind. Of course they are the points that the panel expects in every participant. The following shows some of the qualities that a participant should possess.

Awareness	Team player	Inspiring ability
Assertiveness	Reasoning	Behaviour and interaction
Attitude	Flexible	Open Mindedness
Analytical Skills	Initiative	Way of putting views
Creativity (out of the box thinking)	Patient listening	Leadership
Subject knowledge	Communication	Problem solving
Critical thinking	Confidence	Decision making

Steps during Group Discussion:

1. **Personality manifestation:** The panelists keenly look at signals sent out by your body language and language you speak. Intra personal traits like anger, irritation, frustration, warmth, excitement, defensiveness, competitiveness etc.

2. **Time factor:** You should note the total and individual time carefully. Plan your points accordingly. Sometimes it may be possible that you might not have any time

to keep some good points forth. So it is better to manage the time and plan your points accordingly.

3. **Initiation:** If you are aware of the topic, it is easy for you to break the ice. But one thing that you have to keep in mind is that, if you are starting the topic you should give a brief introduction of the topic so that all those who are unaware of the topic may have some idea of it.

4. **Co-operation:** Cooperate with others and respect their views as well. Help others if they are wrong at some point. Appreciate others' views. This gives an impression that you possess good team building and leadership skills.

5. **Patient Listening:** According to modern psychology, man's greatest desire is to be liked. Listening to other person is one way of showing appreciation. only a good listener is a good speaker. Sometimes it may be possible that the given topic is entirely new for you. In such condition you should allow two or three speakers to speak. In this way you may get an idea of the topic. A group discussion is in fact, an exercise both in speaking and listening.

6. **Be relevant:** Talking trash is worse than remaining silent. But you should note it down that irrelevant speaking is also not advisable and is treated as a negative trait. So try to be relevant without deviating from the topic and beating around the bush.

7. **Accept Criticism:** Unless you are ready to accept criticism, you have no right to criticize other participants. So it is a good quality to be ready that if you are keeping some views in discussion, some or other will definitely oppose them. Moreover it is the part of discussion.

8. **Communication Skills:** They include both verbal and non-verbal communication. You have to be good in expressing yourself with clarity of speech, fluency, proper modulation and good delivery of your statements. You should maintain proper eye contact while speaking with other speaker (s). Your facial expressions should be natural and controlled. Excessive body movements should be avoided as possible. Never try to dominate while using a lot of time for yourself.

9. **Pronunciation:** Be careful about the pronunciation of each and every word you are using in the sentences in discussion. It is possible that you may be thinking some different pronunciation of some words that are pronounced differently. Earn them as possible.

10. **Tongue Twisters:** There are many words that are very difficult to pronounce because of their difficult and different spellings. Practice some tongue twisters available in books and internet. Practice phonetics to be perfect in pronunciation.

11. **Body Language:** If we are trying to make a good impression – both socially and in business – we often smile and hold contact the other person's eyes as we shake their hand. Just by shaking hand or standing in a particular way, we might trigger off old memories in the person we are trying to impress. But if we stand like the back-stabbing colleague who has treated them badly, our advances are likely to be treated as hostile.

EXERCISE

1. What is group discussion?
2. Why group discussion is considered as an important tool to get a job?
3. "Group discussion is an important communication skills needed for technical students". Elaborate it.
4. How group discussion is different from debate?
5. How many types of group discussions are there?
6. How to prepare for group discussion on any topic?
7. What are do's and don'ts of group discussion?
8. Which traits are evaluated during group discussion?
9. Which type of role one should play for getting maximum score in group discussion?
10. Write a short note on importance of group discussion for pharmacy students ?

✸✸✸